The
EVERYTHING
Twins, Triplets, and More Book

Dear Reader:

Finding out I was having twins was certainly a big surprise. After I recovered from the shock, my feelings fluctuated from nauseating despair (or was that morning sickness?) to giddy elation. I was desperately anxious to discover how I'd actually manage to care for two babies simultaneously. At that time, there were very few books that realistically conveyed the experience of a twin pregnancy, much less prepared parents for the challenge of raising multiples once they arrived.

This is the book that I would have wanted to read prior to the birth of my twin daughters. It informs rather than alarms, preparing you to face your future with multiples. First-time parents will be relieved to know that, in some ways, managing more than one is actually easier than singletons of different ages! Established parents will discover how to accommodate the unique demands of multiples while integrating the new additions into their existing lifestyle.

Every aspect of having twins has exceeded my expectations. However, the biggest surprise has been the joy I've experienced along the way. Certainly, my husband and I have seen our share of double drudgery, with hectic days followed by sleepless nights. But as with many things in life, the rewards far outweigh the sacrifices. The love that you give to your multiples will be returned to you exponentially.

Pamela P. Fierro

The EVERYTHING® Series

Editorial

Publishing Director	Gary M. Krebs
Managing Editor	Kate McBride
Copy Chief	Laura M. Daly
Acquisitions Editor	Kate Burgo
Development Editor	Christina MacDonald
Production Editors	Jamie Wielgus
	Bridget Brace
Technical Reviewer	Marcello Pietrantoni, M.D.

Production

Production Director	Susan Beale
Production Manager	Michelle Roy Kelly
Series Designers	Daria Perreault
	Colleen Cunningham
	John Paulhus
Cover Design	Paul Beatrice
	Matt LeBlanc
Layout and Graphics	Colleen Cunningham
	Monica Rhines
Series Cover Artist	Barry Littmann
Interior Illustrator	Eric Andrews

Visit the entire Everything® Series at *www.everything.com*

THE

EVERYTHING®

TWINS, TRIPLETS, and MORE BOOK

From seeing the first sonogram to
coordinating nap times and feedings—
all you need to enjoy your multiples

Pamela Fierro

Adams Media
Avon, Massachusetts

To Brian, my true companion, for loving me no matter what.

An Everything® Series Book.
Everything® and everything.com® are registered trademarks of F+W Publications, Inc.

Published by Adams Media, an F+W Publications Company
57 Littlefield Street, Avon, MA 02322 U.S.A.
www.adamsmedia.com

ISBN: 1-59337-326-0
Printed in the United States of America.

J I H G F E D C B A

Library of Congress Cataloging-in-Publication Data
Fierro, Pamela.
The everything twins, triplets, and more book / Pamela Fierro.
p.   cm.
(Everything series book)
ISBN 1-59337-326-0
1. Multiple birth—Popular works. 2. Multiple pregnancy—Popular works. I. Title. II. Series: Everything series.

RG696.F54 2005
618.2'5--dc22
2005009555

This book is available at quantity discounts for bulk purchases.
For information, please call 1-800-872-5627.

Contents

Acknowledgments

I must accord a special acknowledgement to my two extraordinary daughters, Lauren Marissa and Meredith Rebecca, whose arrival introduced me to the amazing world of twins and multiples.

Thanks to Barb Doyen and Kate Burgo for presenting me with the opportunity to write about this topic. I'd also like to thank the professionals who shared their time and expertise with me: Dr. David G. Oelberg, M.D., Professor of Pediatrics at Eastern Virginia Medical School and Director of the Division of Neonatal-Perinatal Medicine; Robin Elise Weiss, BA, LCCE, ICCE-CPE, CD (DONA), author of *The Everything® Pregnancy Fitness Book* and *The Everything® Getting Pregnant Book*; and my fellow guide writers at About.com. In addition, I am very appreciative of all the mothers of multiples who shared their personal experiences with me, especially Chris Wingard, Denise Anderson, Cindy Mayfield, Suzie Chafin, Mary Ann Magnant, and Marnie Dyer.

Finally, I am eternally grateful to the friends and family members who supported me with prayer and loving care of my children while I worked on this book.

Top Ten Myths and Misconceptions
About Multiples

1. Multiples usually skip a generation.

2. Fraternal twins are always a boy and a girl.

3. Twins with two placentas must be fraternal twins.

4. You have to buy two (or three, or more) of everything for your multiple babies.

5. All multiples must be born by cesarean section.

6. Having two kids close in age is the same as having twins.

7. Having twins is twice as hard, and triplets make it three times as hard, for parents.

8. Identical twins always look exactly alike.

9. It's impossible to breastfeed multiples.

10. You must have taken fertility drugs if you have twins or more.

Foreword

▶ I AM DELIGHTED to introduce a new text by Pamela Fierro written for those unique mothers carrying multiples. This book makes a notable contribution to the body of works on multiple pregnancies and covers areas that many women are concerned about, but which are often covered only superficially by other pregnancy books and professional caregivers. Written with a practical approach, you'll get significant insight on what to expect and critical knowledge about the issues associated with twins, triplets, or greater multiple gestations. The author debunks and explains the myths and misconceptions that surround being pregnant with multiples.

Being pregnant with multiples is an exciting time. There's no doubt this pregnancy will have a big impact on the family as a whole in every way. The babies' arrival will mean changes for everyone, and this book takes you through the necessary steps to prepare. First-time parents will be keenly interested to learn that managing more than one baby is actually easier. Parents who already have other children will learn about the different demands unique to multiples. The author provides a full discussion regarding every aspect of having multiples.

This book is an excellent resource for complex reproductive issues and the obstetrical complications that can occur with multiple gestations. The author provides the reader with a variety of solutions to the problems faced by mothers with a multiples pregnancy and includes plenty of well-documented references for the facts she presents. This book fills a large void in the literature on multiple pregnancies. This is a reference for all couples who struggle to find answers to the most commonly asked questions regarding cutting-edge opinions and technologies, with up-to-date and very comprehensive information on the topics from before conception all the way through birth.

—Marcello Pietrantoni, M.D., F.A.C.O.G., M.P.H.

Introduction

▶ So, you're having multiples! As a parent, you've been gifted with a treasure: a set of twins, triplets, or more—an instant family, so to speak. There's no doubt about it, this will have a big impact on you and the other members of your family. The arrival of the new babies will mean some changes for everyone.

These days, very few multiples make a surprise appearance in the delivery room. Chances are, you have some time to prepare for their entrance into this world. You'll be able to make informed choices along the way, from investing in baby equipment to selecting child care. You'll take the necessary steps to prepare your household and line up assistance so that everyone's needs are met. You'll also be able to prepare yourself physically for the challenges of a multiple pregnancy; by taking good care of yourself, you'll optimize your chances of a healthy outcome for each baby as well as yourself.

Whether you conceived using assistance from reproductive technology or on your own, the news that you're having multiples may have come as quite a shock. Your mind is probably whirling with questions. "How could this happen?" "Why me?" The more you learn about the biology of multiples, the more you'll understand how you came to be in this position. Whether due to science, heredity, or a random coincidence, ultimately multiples are a miracle.

You're likely to experience some negative reactions when you begin to share your news. "Double trouble!" "Triple terror!" "Better you than me!" However, you'll only hear that reaction from people who don't actually have multiples. Talk to the families that have been similarly blessed, and they'll respond with smiles and congratulations. They are the ones who know the true joy and amazement of raising multiples. It's important to seek these people out as a source of reassurance and support.

You may have some ambivalence and anxiety about the situation as well. How will you cope? Can you afford twins or more? Will you need a bigger car or even a bigger home? Health concerns loom large. Suddenly you've been upgraded to a high-risk pregnancy, with vague threats of prolonged bed rest, preterm labor, and complications for your babies. This book will help allay some of your worries.

Identifying and learning about potential problems during pregnancy shouldn't alarm you. Rather, it should be informative. In the event that you encounter problems, you'll be educated about your options and prepared to deal with the consequences. With some extra monitoring and precautions, your chances are quite good for a healthy outcome.

Adjusting your expectations as a parent is an important component of preparing for the arrival of multiples. You'll have to switch your focus from one baby to two or more. It's easy to classify multiples as a set or a group, but you'll quickly realize that each of your children is a distinct personality. Your challenge will be to identify and meet their needs as individuals. It is a fascinating process to watch them develop as unique entities within the context of their bond as twins or multiples.

Having twins, triplets, or higher order multiples is a challenge, but one that reaps huge rewards. They bring a unique dynamic to a family, a special status that sets you apart from families with singletons. Not only are they a blessing to their parents, but they will enjoy lifelong companionship and a special bond with each other.

Chapter 1
The Magic of Multiples

Welcome to the wonderful world of multiples! If you just recently made the discovery that your family is being expanded by twins, triplets, or more, you are probably feeling a bit overwhelmed. You may be curious as to how it came to pass. You may be anxious about how multiples will mesh with your family's lifestyle, and how you will meet the needs of several simultaneous siblings. Having multiples is a truly unique parenting experience, filled with fascination and occasional moments of frustration.

Myths and Mysteries about Multiples

People have long been fascinated by multiple births. Since ancient times, twins have played a role in mythology and legend. In some cultures they are revered; in others they are considered an abomination. Twins are often used symbolically to represent the contrast between good and evil or as a symbol of true companionship.

Multiples in Mythology

A Navajo Indian legend describes two twins, Monster-Slayer and Reared-in-the-Earth, who traveled a secret pollen path to their father, the Sun, and were granted the sacred art of healing through sand painting. In the ancient Mayan culture, the Maize god twins and their sons, the Hero twins, are credited with creation of the human race. The zodiacal constellation of Gemini represents twins Castor and Pollux, inseparable brothers who were willing to share everything, including immortality. In Roman mythology, Romulus and Remus were twins raised by a she-wolf; they grew up to found the city of Rome.

Common Twin Misconceptions

The legendary status of twins has created some interesting misconceptions. Multiples are not identical clones of each other. They are completely unique individuals who happened to be born at the same time. They don't have ESP and can't read each other's minds, although they sometimes finish each other's sentences and often seem to be eerily in tune with each other's thoughts.

Multiples, especially monozygotic or identical twins, make a fascinating case study for the age-old debate of nature versus nurture. Does our genetic makeup determine our personalities and traits, or are we products of our environment? In multiples, researchers can study individuals with both the same genetic composition and shared environment. Participation by twins in research studies helps scientists uncover the causes of medical conditions as well as the development of cures and treatments.

Contrary to popular belief, they are not diminished as individuals simply by being multiples. Some people mistakenly assume that twins or other multiples will be less intelligent, less talented, or otherwise deficient because they share genes. This is absolutely not the case. Research shows no correlation between decreased intelligence or ability and multiple birth.

It's also not true that they can be categorized into opposing groups. In other words, in any given twin set, you can't label one as all good and one as all bad. There's not a "smart one" and a "pretty one." It just doesn't work that way. Unfortunately, sometimes people apply those labels to multiples, and if the children hear such talk often enough as they grow up, they may begin to identify and define themselves according to these views of others.

What's Different about Multiples

By having twins, triplets, or other multiples, you have been granted inclusion into a special class of parents. Although they wouldn't necessarily have asked for this honor, most parents wouldn't trade it for the world. Maybe you have always had a secret fascination with multiples and suspected you would bear them. Or maybe you thought you'd be the last person on earth to have multiples. Either way, this blessing will set you apart from other families and bring a new designation to your identity as a parent.

As a parent of multiples, you'll often hear people say, "Oh, my kids were only eleven months apart. It was just like having twins." There's no easy way—and no good reason—to politely explain to someone that the two situations are nothing alike. It's easiest just to smile and nod agreeably.

Having multiples is extraordinary. If you gathered a group of one hundred parents, only two or three would be able to claim multiples. For the rest of your life, you are guaranteed to get a reaction when you talk about your children. Gasps of "Oh!" "Wow!" "Lucky you!" and "Better you than me!" are common responses when you tell someone you have multiples.

Some people might wonder what the big deal is about twins and multiples. Plenty of families have lots of kids, right? What makes it so different to have a few of them at once? There are many ways that having two, three, or more babies at the same time is different than having the same number of singletons. In some ways it makes family life easier, but in others it makes things much more complicated. No matter how close in age singletons may be, the fact remains that they were born one at a time. Their parents had at least nine months to prepare for the arrival of the next child. The organizational challenges of simultaneously meeting the needs of multiple newborns are simply more demanding.

The Impact of Birth Order

Birth order has a tremendous impact on the structure of families. Not only does it contribute to the personality development of each individual child, but it also sets the standard for how each child is treated. Older children have more freedom, but likewise more responsibility, because their advanced age makes them developmentally capable of handling it. Younger children benefit from interaction with their older siblings.

Multiples, on the other hand, lack the defined roles created by birth order. Being the same age, and generally of equal status within the family, there is no formalized structure for establishing order. The effort to create and reinvent a pecking order can generate ongoing tension for the family as the parents seek to intervene.

The Group Dynamic

Outsiders may look at your duo, trio, or higher order multiples and see two, three, or more kids. What they don't realize is that in addition to having these individual children, as a parent of multiples you also have to contend with a group dynamic. With multiples, parents don't simply have an extra child or two. The group dynamic adds an entirely new element. You know the old saying, "Two heads are better than one?" Working in conjunction with each other, a group of multiples is easily more daring, more creative, and more clever than any individual child on his or her own.

The companionship and cooperation of their same-age siblings often incites behavior that exceeds an individual child's limits. Together, multiples will invent more schemes, attempt more stunts, and create more messes. There is power in numbers, and managing that power is one of the biggest challenges that parents of multiples face.

Playing Fair

Another unique challenge is maintaining equality among multiples. It's often a struggle for parents of twins or more to ensure that each child gets his or her fair share; whether it is time, attention, or material goods, it is difficult (if not impossible) to always dole out an equitable portion. Life is simply not fair. Unfortunately, you can't convince multiples of that fact, and as a parent you can never quit striving to make it so! Soothing jealousy and stifling competition is a constant battle for parents until multiples mature to an age where they can accept and appreciate the differences among them.

ALERT!

Some parents of multiples find it a challenge to teach their children principles of accountability because the twins, triplets, or more are accustomed to sharing joint responsibility with their co-multiples. Frequently rewarded and disciplined as a group, they share blame, as well as credit, without individual accountability.

The Bond They Share

The bond between a set of multiples is unique. Beginning even before birth, it is one of the longest and most enduring interpersonal relationships that a human being can have. It surpasses that of regular siblings. The intensity of this relationship often makes multiples the best of friends one moment and bitter enemies the next.

As a parent, you'll have a unique opportunity to watch your multiples' bond grow and develop from the very beginning. You'll have responsibility for nurturing each child as an individual within the context of their unique relationship to their co-multiples. It's never too early to start thinking about how you'll accomplish that balance.

Share and Share Alike

All members of a family have to learn to share to get along. But multiples share more than most siblings. Beginning in the womb, they share space and, sometimes, a placenta. Most share a birthday. Infant multiples may share a crib, the milk from their mother's breasts, and most of their clothing.

Despite their parents' best efforts to endow them with ownership, multiples will most likely battle for custody over every toy and plaything that crosses their path. However, they'll generously share every germ and virus that comes their way. Of course, they'll share lots of fun, too, commemorating milestones and making happy memories together as they grow up. As playmates, they will have access to instant stimulation and constant companionship, often relieving parents of the burden of providing entertainment for their children.

Give and Take

Whether it is a parent's attention, the right to be first, or sole ownership of a plaything they're after, multiples can be extremely competitive with one another. Many multiples are able to channel their competitive natures into achievement when they grow older, excelling in sports or academics.

Sometimes the dynamic between a pair of multiples is one of compensating, rather than competing. Where one is lacking in a character attribute or skill, the other will step up to the plate. For example, many multiples exhibit delays in language development because the twin with stronger language skills will do most of the talking for her weaker sibling, communicating for both of them.

QUESTION?

Do identical twins have a closer bond than fraternal twins?
While the scientific community might argue that shared DNA makes them more compatible, the consensus among parents of multiples seems to indicate that this has no bearing on their relationship. Sometimes identical twins don't get along simply because they are too similar, while fraternal multiples craft an incredibly close bond due to their shared environment.

Famous Multiples

Now that you know you're having a set of your own, you'll start seeing multiples everywhere! There have been many well-known multiples throughout history, as well as famous parents of twins, triplets, or more.

Twins on TV

Multiples have had starring roles in many television shows—just look at the surprise birth of twins adopted by Monica and Chandler in the final episode of *Friends*; Carla, the wisecracking waitress on the show *Cheers*, had twins on that show; and twins were also born to characters on *The Nanny* and *Welcome Back, Kotter*. There are twins among the seven siblings on *Seventh Heaven*. Teenage twins, Brandon and Brenda Walsh, led the cast of characters on *Beverly Hills 90210*.

Some TV parents have twins in real life. Ray Romano plays a dad of twins on his show, *Everyone Loves Raymond*, and also raises twin boys off the show. A sense of humor comes in handy when you're a parent of multiples! Fred MacMurray was the grandfather of triplets on *My Three Sons* and the father of twin girls in real life. Both Patricia Richardson, the mom on *Home Improvement*, and Meredith Baxter-Birney of *Family Ties* have a set of fraternal twins.

The "Six Million Dollar Man" didn't have six million dollar kids, but actor Lee Majors does have twin boys. Another TV tough guy, *Bonanza*'s Lorne Greene, was also a father of twins.

Sometimes television personalities grow up and are blessed with multiples. Michael J. Fox and his wife, Tracy Pollan, have twin girls. Richard Thomas, AKA John Boy Walton, has triplets. Ron Howard, beloved as Opie on *The Andy Griffith Show* and Richie Cunningham on *Happy Days*, became the father of twin girls. Other TV actors who are parents of multiples include:

- Chuck Norris
- Ed Asner
- Christine Lahti
- Steve Harvey
- Peri Gilpin
- Jane Seymour
- Cybill Shepherd

Probably the most famous TV twins are Mary-Kate and Ashley Olsen, who got their start playing a single character, Michelle, on the television series *Full House* in 1987. They went on to build a media empire with countless movie and video features, music CDs, a clothing line, toys, and other merchandise.

Twins in the Movies

Fascination with twins has been a theme throughout movie history. Common plots include twins trying to kill each other, competing for romantic interests, or becoming reunited after being separated at birth. Happily, real life with multiples is not nearly that dramatic!

Several movie actors are twins, or have twins. Tough-guy actors Robert deNiro and Al Pacino both fathered twins. Mia Farrow has fraternal twins with Andre Previn. Oscar winner Marcia Gay Harden gave birth to twins in 2004. Superstar Julia Roberts bore twins in late 2004. Classic star Jimmy Stewart was the father of twin girls. Movie hunks Mel Gibson and Denzel Washington are both fathers of twins.

The Terminator's Linda Hamilton has a twin sister. Likewise, Scarlett Johansson, Isabella Rossellini, Ashton Kutcher, Kiefer Sutherland, and Jon Lovitz all have twin siblings. Actor Andy Garcia was born as a conjoined twin; his stillborn brother was surgically removed right after birth.

Twins in Space

Several twins and their parents have traveled in space. The first twin in space was Charles Duke. He was part of the early space program in the late 1960s and 1970s, piloting several of the Apollo missions to the moon. Twin brothers Mark and Scott Kelly were both accepted into NASA's astronaut training program in the late 1990s; they are the only set of twins to travel in space, although not at the same time. They participated in space shuttle missions in 1999 and 2001, respectively. Several other astronauts are fathers of twins, including Gerald Carr and Donald Pettit, and Carlos Noriega has triplets.

FACT

Jim Bunning, a baseball Hall of Fame player best known for pitching a perfect game in 1964, is the father of two sets of twins.

Multiples in Sports

Perhaps due to their competitive natures, many multiples excel in sports. Twins and triplets are found among the leading athletes in many sports, including football, baseball, basketball, and soccer. Perhaps one of the best known pairs is Tiki and Ronde Barber, professional football players who often compete against each other on opposing teams. Several sets of female twins are successful professional soccer players, including

- Julie and Nancy Augustyniak
- Lorrie and Ronnie Fair
- Jacqui and Skylar Little
- Jennifer and Margaret Tietjen

Several fathers of higher order multiples have found a home in Major League Baseball. Dennis Cook, Luis Gonzalez, Dave Righetti, and Phil Hiatt are all fathers of triplets. Doug Strange has quads and Melvin Mora is the father of quintuplets.

Champion parents of twins can be found in every realm of sports. Boxer Muhammad Ali and cyclist Lance Armstrong are both fathers of twin girls. Tennis champion Ivan Lendl and soccer superstar Pele also fathered twins. Vanetta Flowers, the first African-American to win a gold medal in the Olympics, had twin boys after her bobsled victory.

Quite a few multiples found success in the 2004 Olympics in Athens, Greece, perhaps inspired by the twin mascots of the games. (Athena and

Phevos represented the Greek deities Athena, the goddess of wisdom and patron of Athens, and Apollo, the god of light and music.) Mike and Bob Bryan, the top doubles team in the world, represented the United States in tennis. Twin brothers Paul and Morgan Hamm led the men's gymnastic team to a silver medal; Paul found further success winning an individual gold in the all-around competition.

Twins in Music

Imagine being sung a lullaby by Dave Matthews, James Taylor, Bruce Hornsby, Bing Crosby, Nat "King" Cole, or Julio Iglesias! These talented crooners are all fathers of twins. In classical music, Johann Sebastian Bach was the father of twins; in addition, his own father had a twin brother.

Some of the biggest talents in music history are twinless twins. Elvis Presley's twin, Jesse, was born stillborn. Flamboyant performer Liberace and teen pop idol Justin Timberlake both lost their twins at birth.

Twin singing sensations are found in every genre of music. Fraternal twins Robin and Maurice Gibb joined with older brother Barry to form the pop and disco group the Bee Gees. Ian and Kevin Greenlaw are identical twin opera singers. Teen star Aaron Carter has a twin sister. Evan and Jaron Lowenstein are twin brothers who perform together as pop singers. Loretta Lynn's twin daughters, Peggy and Patsy, followed in their mother's footsteps as country singers. Benji and Joel Madden found fame on MTV with their band, Good Charlotte. Twin brothers Charlie and Craig Reid are The Proclaimers, a Scottish band.

Twins in the News

There are a surprising number of parents of twins in the television news industry. They can be found at all the major networks. Bob Woodruff is a reporter at ABC and the father of twin girls. Lou Dobbs, anchor of a popular financial series at CNN, is also the father of twin girls. Soledad O'Brien, anchor of a morning show on CNN, had twin boys in 2004. Jane Pauley, a longtime newswoman at NBC, along with husband Gary Trudeau, the author of the *Doonesbury* comic, have fraternal twins. Joan Lunden had fraternal twins via surrogacy after leaving ABC. Marc Mancuso of The Weather Channel is the father of twin girls.

Other Famous Multiples

President George W. Bush has fraternal twin daughters who graduated from college in 2004. He's had several fellow twin parents in his cabinet, including U.S. Energy Secretary Spence Abraham. Other world leaders, both past and present, have been parents of twins. King Louis IV of France, American Vice President Nelson Rockefeller, British Prime Minister Margaret Thatcher, Cleopatra, and King Hussein of Jordan had twins, and it is rumored that Abraham Lincoln illegitimately fathered a set of twins.

Children's author Beverly Cleary is the mother of twins, while fellow author Avi has a twin sister who gave him the nickname he uses as a pseudonym. William Shakespeare fathered a set of boy-girl twins. Scottish poet Robert Burns had two sets of twins. Twin sisters Ann Landers and Abby Van Buren wrote competing advice columns in newspapers around the world.

Chapter 2

An Introduction to Zygosity

One of the first and most common questions that you will be asked about your multiples is "Are they identical or fraternal?" Although most people understand that these are the two basic types of twins, some members of the general public truly have no idea what these terms really describe. Twin type (this term refers to all multiples, not just twins) has very little to do with appearance, and everything to do with the originating relationship of the individuals. It's based on zygosity.

What Is Zygosity?

Most people are familiar with the terms *identical* and *fraternal*, but the categorizations don't represent twin type as accurately as the more scientific classifications of zygosity. Scientifically speaking, there are two basic types of multiples. Monozygotic, or identical, multiples are the result of a single zygote, or fertilized egg, while dizygotic (or multizygotic) multiples form from two or more zygotes. These multiples are commonly termed *fraternal*. All twins fit into one of these categories. Triplets, quadruplets, and other higher order multiples may be one or the other, or even a combination of both. For example, two children in a set of triplets may be monozygotic while the third is dizygotic. Twin typing, or determining zygosity, means figuring out which of these two types of multiples you have.

To understand zygosity, you have to start at the very beginning: conception. It starts when a woman's ovary releases an egg, or oocyte, into her fallopian tube and it travels toward the uterus. This process is called ovulation, and happens monthly. Along the way, sperm released by a male during sexual intercourse try to intercept the oocyte. If a sperm is able to penetrate, the egg becomes fertilized. The fertilized oocyte continues its journey to the uterus, dividing and combining cells to form a zygote. It implants in the uterus and begins to grow into a baby. But variations in the process can produce multiples—twins, triplets, or more. Zygosity not only defines twin type, but can give parents valuable insight into their multiples' origin.

QUESTION?

Why is it important to understand zygosity?
Determining the zygosity of your multiples is significant on several levels. First, it's nice to have an answer when people ask whether your multiples are fraternal or identical! It's also helpful to understand how and why you became pregnant with multiples. But, more importantly, determining zygosity is important in identifying certain medical issues associated with twinning.

Dizygotic Twins

Sometimes during the ovulation process, the ovaries are prompted to release multiple eggs. There are many reasons for this occurrence. A normal female body has two ovaries, one on the left side and one on the right. Both contain thousands of eggs. Generally the ovaries take turns ovulating, but occasionally they will each release an egg in a single cycle. Some women have a genetic tendency to hyperovulate, or release numerous eggs every month. Other women might release multiple eggs on an occasional basis due to hormonal fluctuations. Sometimes hormones are influenced medically, by taking drugs such as birth control pills or fertility enhancements such as Clomid or Pergonal. But they can also be impacted by a woman's age (older women tend to release multiple eggs more often than younger women), or by lifestyle.

Dizygotic twins are conceived if two eggs are fertilized by sperm (*di* meaning two and *zygotic* referring to the fertilized egg, or zygote). If both zygotes implant in the uterus, you've got twins! Likewise, three zygotes produce triplets and four would be quadruplets. Generally, even higher order multiples that are born of separate zygotes are all referred to as dizygotic, although a more correct term would be multizygotic.

Dizygotic Defined

Dizygotic twins are essentially siblings that happen to be born at the same time. They are each formed from a separate egg and a separate sperm. Just as related children within a family have a variety of appearances and characteristics based on the combination of genetic traits they inherit from their parents, dizygotic twins can also be very alike or very different. They can be boys, girls, or one of each.

When people talk about twins being hereditary or skipping a generation, they are referring to dizygotic twins. Women with a gene for hyperovulation are more likely to conceive twins since they routinely release multiple eggs. Their daughters have an increased chance of having twins as well, if they inherit the gene. However, if a woman gives birth to a son, his impact on the twinning process is irrelevant, as men do not have ovaries or ovulate. However, his daughter may inherit the hyperovulation tendency and produce twin grandchildren, thus causing the gene to "skip" a generation.

Causes of Dizygotic Twinning

Many other interesting characteristics influence dizygotic twinning. A woman's chances of conceiving dizygotic twins increase when:

- She's had a previous multiple pregnancy.
- She's over age forty-five.
- She's already had several other children.
- She is a dizygotic twin herself, or her mother or maternal grandmother was a twin.
- She has irregular sexual intercourse.
- She conceives shortly after discontinuing birth control pills. (This is not recommended due to the risk of birth defects.)

The radical rise in the multiple birth rate since the latter part of the twentieth century is mostly observed among dizygotic multiples. It's generally attributed to the impact of advancing maternal age as women put off childbearing until they're older, which heightens their chance of releasing duplicate eggs. The increase in assisted reproduction and fertility enhancements is another contributing factor.

Monozygotic Twins

As opposed to dizygotic twins, monozygotics form from a single zygote. (*Mono* means one.) For reasons yet to be exactly determined by science, a single fertilized egg sometimes splits into two individual zygotes; both begin the process of dividing and combining cells to form embryos, resulting in two babies.

ESSENTIAL

Dizygotic twins generally outnumber monozygotics by about two to one. Interestingly, monozygotic twinning rates remain steady despite an overall increase in multiple birth. Further, monozygotic rates are the same across populations; you're equally likely to have identical twins whether you're Japanese or African.

No one knows exactly what causes an egg to split. Several theories have been formulated, but none are accepted as fact. Some scientists believe that it is related to the age of the egg, while others suggest that an enzyme in certain sperm is the cause. But no one knows for sure, and monozygotic twinning remains one of the great magical mysteries of life. A zygote can split more than once. Some triplets, quadruplets, and one documented case of quintuplets, the Dionne sisters, are monozygotic.

Because they have formed from a single zygote, monozygotic twins share the same genetic makeup. Since many human physical characteristics are determined by genetics, monozygotic twins may share a remarkable resemblance. This is why the term "identical" is a common way to describe them. However, environmental influences also affect appearance, so no two twins are ever exactly alike.

Monozygotic twins are always of the same sex. The only exception is an extremely rare condition where a chromosomal abnormality in male monozygotic twins results in the loss of a Y chromosome in one of them, producing a female afflicted with Turner's syndrome, or "45,X."

FIGURE 2-1
Egg Splitting
Chart

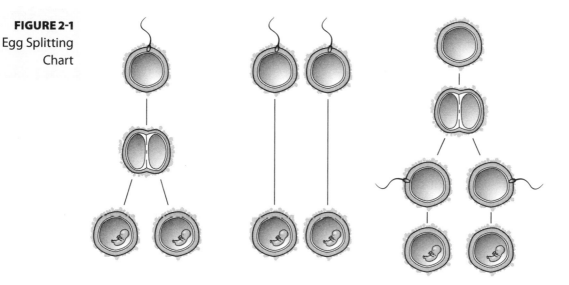

▲ Monozygotic (identical) twins form from a single egg that splits after fertilization. Dizygotic (fraternal) multiples result when more than one egg is fertilized. Polar body twins are the result of a single ova that splits prior to fertilization.

Other Zygosity Variations

Although monozygotic and dizygotic are the two accepted categories of twinship, there are some subtypes that deserve mention. You may or may not be able to determine whether your multiples fit into one of these categories, but they are interesting to consider.

Polar Body Twins

You may have heard of a third type of twinning. Usually this refers to polar body twinning, also known as "half-identical" twins. It's more of a theory than a scientifically accepted fact, but it can provide a tidy explanation for dizygotic twins with a strong resemblance. A polar body is a small cell within the egg that divides off and usually degenerates and dies after fertilization. If, for some reason, the polar body divides off prematurely from the egg, it may also become fertilized by a sperm and develop as an embryo. No one is sure why or how it happens, and it appears to be very rare.

Developing from a single egg but separate sperm, these twins share about 75 percent of their genotypes: 50 percent from their mother, but only 25 percent from their father. They would be more "identical," or similar in appearance, than dizygotic twins but less so than monozygotics. At this time, there isn't a way to definitively determine the existence of polar body twinning; zygosity testing services that analyze DNA do not include polar body testing in their results.

FACT

Popular television and movie twins Mary-Kate and Ashley Olsen are rumored to be polar body twins. The media repeatedly confirms that the actresses are fraternal, yet their remarkable resemblance is undeniable.

Dizygotic Variances

Although polar body twinning is considered an alternate twin type, other categories are merely subsets or special types of either monozygotic or dizygotic twinning. Among dizygotic twins, two unique divergences have been identified.

Superfetation occurs when a second egg is inadvertently released in a subsequent reproductive cycle despite the fertilization of the first. The result is multiples that are conceived at different times, up to twenty-four days apart. Superfetation may account for discrepancies in fetal size and development in dizygotic multiples. If confirmed during the pregnancy, the "older" baby may be delivered days or even weeks before his twin to promote optimal gestational well-being.

Superfecundation, on the other hand, describes a situation where dizygotic twins have different fathers. It happens when an ovulating woman has intercourse with multiple partners within a short time frame. Two eggs are fertilized by sperm from different men. Several cases of superfecundation have been identified and confirmed by DNA testing, including a case in Europe in the 1970s where the babies were of different races.

Mirror Image Twins

Mirror image twins are an example of a special type of monozygotic twins. About 23 percent of monozygotic twins are classified as "mirror image," in that they exhibit reversed asymmetry in certain physical characteristics. For example, hair whorls rotate in opposite directions, moles or birthmarks are featured on opposite sides of the body, or the two have opposite hand preferences. In very rare cases, vital organs may develop on opposite sides of their bodies.

There's no way to diagnostically confirm mirror image twins, except by observation of their features. It's believed that mirror image twinning occurs due to a delayed split, about a week after fertilization, when the developing embryo has a clearly established right and left side. Mirror image twins generally share a placenta and other characteristics of monozygotic twins.

Conjoined Twins

Conjoined twins are a type of monozygotic multiples, originating from a single zygote that splits into two. However, they take their time splitting apart, with the consequence that they do not entirely separate, and begin to develop with connected tissue or organs. With an increase in media attention focused on conjoined twins, it may seem that they are becoming more common. However, conjoined twins are an extremely rare type of monozygotic twins, representing only 1 in 50,000 pregnancies.

Although some conjoined twins live into old age, most are afflicted by health complications due to strain on their shared organs. It is estimated that about 50 percent of conjoined twins are stillborn, and many more do not survive more than a few days after birth. Even with a minimal connection, it is difficult for conjoined twins to lead a normal life.

Modern medical technology makes surgical separation of conjoined twins an increasingly viable option, even when vital organs are shared. Recent success stories like the Egyptian brothers Ahmed and Mohamed Ibrahim, Guatemalan sisters Maria Teresa and Mara de Jesus Quiej-Alvarez, and Filipino brothers Carl and Clarence Aguirre provide hope for a healthy future. (See Chapter 12 for more information on conjoined twins.)

Twin Typing in Utero

So how will you know what kind of multiples you have? In the past, some multiples never knew the truth about their origin. But as modern technology provides new ways to reveal the clues, conclusive information is more accessible. In some cases, doctors can even identify zygosity before the babies ever arrive.

Using Ultrasound

The babies' arrangement in the womb may provide some clues about their zygosity, although the signs aren't always conclusive. First, an ultrasound examination can provide a tip-off: the sex of the babies. If they are of opposite sex, they are obviously dizygotic. However, if the gender cannot be determined, or if all babies are of the same gender, they could be either monozygotic or dizygotic.

Placenta Analysis

Doctors can also use ultrasound to examine the placenta. Studying the placenta can be helpful in determining zygosity because the placental structure of monozygotic and dizygotic twins sometimes varies.

In any pregnancy, single or multiple, the fertilized egg travels to the uterus and implants in the uterine wall; from this point it is referred to as an embryo. The process may take several days. About a week after fertilization, the placenta begins to form along the inner wall of the uterus. Dizygotic multiples will implant individually in the uterus and develop individual placentas. Monozygotic twins, on the other hand, may follow one of several courses depending on when the zygote splits. If the split occurs early, within four days post conception, monozygotics will act much as dizygotics; they'll implant separately and, at least initially, have two distinct placentas. Early-forming monozygotics can be indistinguishable from dizygotics.

ALERT!

Determining zygosity before birth is tricky since the evidence is often inconclusive. Unless doctors can definitively identify two fetuses of the same gender with a shared placenta and a shared sac, they can't be sure whether the multiples are dizygotic or monozygotic. To complicate matters, two placentas may fuse together over time, appearing as a single entity.

The majority of monozygotics, about 68 percent, experience the split between four and eight days post fertilization. They will share a placenta and be enclosed within a shared chorion (the outer layer of the sac that contains a fetus), but will develop individually within separate and distinct amnions (the inner membrane surrounding the sac of amniotic fluid). These twins are referred to as monochorionic monozygotics. A small percentage of monozygotic twins, less than 2 percent, split after the amnion forms on or about day eight, and develop jointly within a shared amnion. Monoamnionic multiples will also share a single placenta and chorion. Doctors can often use ultrasound technology to determine the number of placentas and the structure of the chorion and amnion by identifying the membrane separating them. The absence of a distinguishing membrane may indicate monozygotic twins.

FIGURE 2-2
Chart of
Membranes

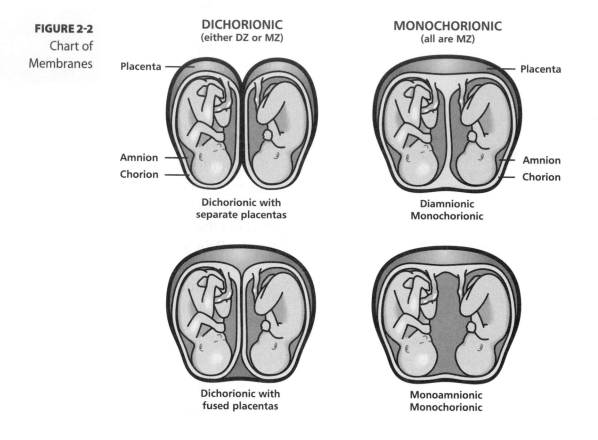

DICHORIONIC
(either DZ or MZ)

MONOCHORIONIC
(all are MZ)

Placenta

Placenta

Amnion
Chorion

Amnion
Chorion

**Dichorionic with
separate placentas**

**Diamnionic
Monochorionic**

**Dichorionic with
fused placentas**

**Monoamnionic
Monochorionic**

▲ Depending on when the egg splits, monozygotic twins will have two separate placentas (dichorionic) that may or may not fuse together. Or they may share a single placenta (monochorionic) but have individual amniotic sacs. Monoamniotic twins are encased in a single sac.

After Birth

Sometimes you can't determine the zygosity of multiples until after they are born. After your babies are delivered, your physician may examine the placenta(s) visually or send them to a laboratory for pathological testing.

Most monochorionic monozygotics are identified by laboratory analysis of the placenta after birth.

In the meantime, your babies may confirm or confound your suspicions by their similarities or dissimilarities. Even monozygotics may appear radically different due to their birth experience (perhaps one was a breech delivery) or factors in the uterine environment. On the other hand, some dizygotics have a strong resemblance as infants, which fades as they grow older.

What if you still don't know for sure? If you have same-sex babies that look alike but had two separate placentas, they could be either dizygotic or monozygotic. If you want to know the truth, further testing is required. Sometimes a simple blood test will reveal the secret; if the babies have different blood types, they are dizygotic. But if they share the same blood type, you'll have to take the next step and pursue a DNA test.

In most cases, doctors won't routinely order DNA testing to determine zygosity, and insurance won't cover the costs. Fortunately, several private companies now offer twin-type testing services. The process is fairly simple, the results are usually conclusive, and the cost is minimal; several companies offer the test for less than $500.

ESSENTIAL

Because twins and other multiples provide scientists with such a rich resource for research, there is great interest in studying them. Many research studies will cover the cost of zygosity testing for participating multiples. It's one way to unlock the secret of your multiples' origin, while helping scientists unravel the secrets of the universe!

DNA testing determines zygosity by comparing cell samples from each child. Monozygotic twins, evolving from a single gene set, will have comparable samples. Dizygotic multiples, on the other hand, will exhibit differences in their DNA, since each child inherited a unique genetic package from their parents.

Chapter 3

Supertwins: Triplets and More

While twins have become fairly commonplace in our society, triplets and higher order multiples remain relatively rare. Nearly everyone knows a twin or a family with a set of twins in their genealogy. But many people live their entire lives without ever crossing paths with a quadruplet. Discovering that you're about to be responsible for so many babies can be quite daunting! Each additional baby that you welcome into this world represents an increase: in risk, in challenge, but also in blessing.

What Are Supertwins?

The term *supertwins* is used to refer to multiples of three, four, or more. Another term that is commonly used is *higher order multiples*. More descriptive names are assigned to specifically designate the number of babies:

- **Three babies:** Triplets
- **Four babies:** Quadruplets (quads)
- **Five babies:** Quintuplets (quints)
- **Six babies:** Sextuplets
- **Seven babies:** Septuplets
- **Eight babies:** Octuplets
- **Nine babies:** Nonuplets
- **Ten babies:** Decaplets

Higher order multiples are conceived like anyone else, when a sperm meets an egg. Most supertwins are multizygotic, meaning that each individual embryo starts as a single egg-and-sperm combination. Sometimes a pair of individuals within the multiple set will be monozygotic and the rest will be dizygotic. In rare situations, the entire multiple set is monozygotic, the result of a fertilized egg splitting multiple times.

FIGURE 3-1
Supertwins
Zygosity
Permutations

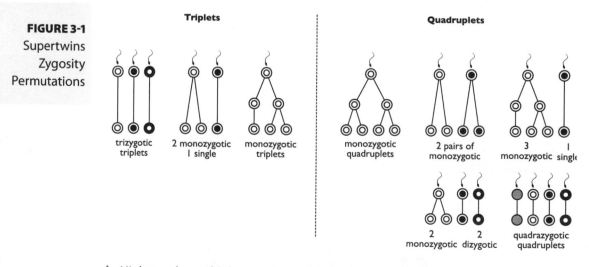

▲ Higher order multiples may be multizygotic, monozygotic, or a combination.

There's no doubt about it. If you're expecting triplets, quadruplets, or more, you've joined a rather elite club of parents. The birth rate for higher order multiples (triplets and more) jumped 380 percent between 1971 and 1995. However, despite this increase, they remain a relatively rare event. Take a look at the statistics:

- Naturally occurring triplet births occur in approximately 1 per 8,500 births.
- Naturally occurring quadruplet births happen only once per 600,000 births.
- The odds of having quintuplets in non-assisted conceptions are 1 in approximately 54,000,000.
- In 2002, about 2,000 sets of triplets and 100 sets of quadruplets were born in the United States.
- Triplets and above represented less than two-tenths of 1 percent of all live births in the United States in 2002.

How did you get so lucky? If you played the lottery with the same odds, you'd likely be a big winner!

Reproductive Technology and Supertwins

Much of the rise in supertwin birthrates over the last thirty years is attributed to advances in reproductive technology. New techniques and procedures increase the ability to produce viable pregnancies. Elizabeth Noble, author of *Having Twins and More*, estimates that three-fourths of higher order multiples are the result of assisted conceptions.

FACT

In March 2004, a Texas woman delivered quadruplet boys that were actually two sets of monozygotic twins. The odds of simultaneously having two sets of monozygotics are estimated at 1 in 11 million births.

Fertility Drugs

Treatment for infertility takes many forms, depending on a couple's specific needs and issues. Fertility-enhancing drugs are often the first step for couples. Prescription drugs, such as Clomid (clomiphene citrate) or Pergonal (human menopausal gonadotropin), manipulate a woman's hormones to induce and regulate ovulation. Sometimes the drugs cause hyperovulation, or the release of multiple eggs. This increases the odds of more than one egg becoming fertilized, and a resulting multizygotic multiple pregnancy.

Although the chances of conceiving twins while taking Clomid are estimated at about 6 percent, the drug is not generally associated with an increased risk of higher order multiples. However, often more powerful drugs are employed when Clomid fails to produce a pregnancy. These can have an extreme impact on ovulation, generating the release of numerous eggs, which, if fertilized, lead to the development of many fetuses. Several recent cases of sextuplets and septuplets are attributed to this type of fertility treatment.

The ART of Reproduction

Assisted reproductive technology (or ART) is the collective term used to describe procedures that involve manipulation of both a female egg and male sperm outside of the female body. There are several approaches that are used, depending on the cause of the infertility issue:

- **In vitro fertilization (IVF):** Eggs are harvested from the mother's ovaries and combined with sperm in a laboratory. (*In vitro* is Latin for "in glass.") The fertilized eggs—or embryos—are placed into the woman's uterus.
- **Gamete intrafallopian transfer (GIFT):** GIFT is similar to IVF, but the eggs are fertilized inside the woman's body rather than outside. The mother's eggs are removed from her ovaries and placed in her fallopian tube along with sperm from the father.
- **Zygote intrafallopian transfer (ZIFT):** ZIFT is a combination of GIFT and IVT. It is also known as tubal embryo transfer. Eggs are fertilized in the lab, then placed in the mother's fallopian tube (rather than the uterus, as in IVF).

In order to enhance the chances of conception, reproductive specialists often transfer multiple eggs or zygotes with the assumption that not all of the eggs will implant in the uterus and be a viable pregnancy. The practice has become a source of controversy because of the increased number of risky multiple births that have resulted. Today it is generally considered inadvisable to transfer more than two or three embryos. Laws regulating the number of embryos have been passed in Europe, and are under review in the United States.

Fertility treatment drastically increases your chances of having multiples. In natural conception, the odds of having multiples are about 1 in 80. Taking fertility drugs ups the odds to 1 in 20, while in vitro fertilization (IVF) results in 1 multiple conception out of every 5 pregnancies.

What about Monozygotics?

Limiting the number of embryos reduces the chance of dizygotic multiples, but it doesn't rule out multiples completely. An interesting relationship has been observed between monozygotic twins and ART. Studies indicate that egg splitting occurs in about 3 percent of assisted pregnancies. One theory proposes that the delay in the zygote's growth and implantation gives it more time to split, but the cause remains as much a mystery as spontaneous incidence of monozygotic twinning.

Whether by uncontrolled ovulation stimulation or overzealous embryo transfers, clearly reproductive technology has resulted in an increase in higher order multiples. Multiple birth is actually considered a complication of reproductive treatment, not the primary goal. Nevertheless, as a result, many previously infertile couples now find themselves the parents of triplets, quadruplets, or more.

Extreme Supertwins

While many animals give birth to litters, the human body is designed to bear only one baby at a time. Generally, two are easily sustained, but every additional baby pushes the situation to an extreme as competition for space and resources increases.

In recent years mothers have given birth to extreme supertwins like sextuplets, septuplets, and even octuplets. Higher order multiples such as these are not a new phenomenon, but their ability to survive has only been established in recent years as medical technology has grown to accommodate the extreme stresses of pregnancy and prematurity.

The first recorded set of surviving quintuplets was born in Canada in 1934. The identical Dionne quintuplets—Annette, Yvonne, Cecile, Marie Rein, and Emilie—became wards of the province of Ontario and were unfortunately turned into a public spectacle.

FACT

The Dionne quints are one example of less than 100 recorded spontaneous quintuplet births. Since the 1960s, less than twenty sets of quints have been conceived without the influence of fertility enhancement.

Although many septuplet pregnancies have occurred, the McCaughey septuplets, born in Iowa in 1997, were the first set where all seven babies survived. They are an example of higher order multiples conceived with the use of powerful fertility drugs. Since their birth, another set was born in Saudi Arabia in 1998, and octuplets were born later that year in Texas. Unfortunately, one of those babies died shortly after birth.

Special Medical Considerations

For many supertwins, merely being born seems a miraculous event. The struggle for survival in the womb puts a strain on both the mother's and babies' health. Each additional baby increases the demands on the mother's physical ability to provide sufficient space and nutrients for everyone.

A supertwin pregnancy requires careful monitoring, and often, more intense medical intervention.

Multiple Challenges for the Mother

Many conditions of pregnancy are intensified in mothers of higher order multiples. Each additional baby contributes to the hormonal fluctuations raging within her body. These hormones that control pregnancy cause many of the typical symptoms such as mood swings, cravings, fatigue, and nausea; the increased levels of these hormones in a mother carrying three, four, or more babies are likely to intensify her experience of the symptoms.

Perhaps the biggest concern in higher order multiple birth is preterm labor. Because of the risk, many mothers of higher order multiples experience more medical intervention. While a twin mother may be able to avoid bed rest or hospitalization during her pregnancy, it is more common for mothers of triplets or quadruplets to require treatment to prevent preterm labor. It is virtually assured that mothers of quintuplets and higher will spend time in the hospital prior to delivery.

QUESTION?

Why are higher order multiples more likely to be born too early?
The average uterus is designed to accommodate about ten pounds of baby. Supertwins usually weigh only half of the average birth weight of their singleton counterparts, but their combined weight easily overwhelms the capacity of the uterus. The risk increases exponentially with each additional baby.

Every pregnancy experience is different, and not every mother of supertwins will have a complicated pregnancy. However, increased tendencies for many complications exist. For example:

- Morning sickness and nausea in early pregnancy may be intensified, leading to improper nutrition and dehydration.
- Iron-deficiency anemia is more common and severe.

- Mothers of higher order multiples are two to three times more likely to have gestational diabetes.
- Complications from the placenta, such as placenta previa or abruptio placentae, are more likely to occur.
- One in three mothers of multiples will contract preeclampsia or pregnancy-induced hypertension, raising her blood pressure to dangerously unhealthy levels.
- Virtually all mothers of multiples higher than triplets will have to deliver by cesarean section, which carries an increased risk of infection, blood loss, and complications, and generally requires a longer recuperation period.

If you're expecting higher order multiples, it is vital that you receive prenatal care from a physician experienced with your situation. Simply having delivered twins is not sufficient experience for treating a woman expecting three, four, or more babies. Obstetricians and perinatologists that specialize in higher order multiples are most accessible in large cities or teaching hospitals, but they are becoming more common as the multiple birth rate increases.

In addition, you should plan to receive care from a hospital with a Level III maternity division. This designation provides assurance that the facility is prepared to meet the needs of high-risk obstetrical patients and can treat the full range of newborn afflictions once your babies are born. Some mothers choose to receive care in another city or even another state in order to ensure the best possible treatment in the event of complications.

Risks to the Babies

The biggest single risk for higher order multiples is premature birth. Without sufficient opportunity to develop in utero, premature babies are at risk for numerous complications and disabilities. Some are apparent at birth, as severely premature infants struggle to maintain the basic operation of life. Other consequences don't manifest themselves until later in life, as the children develop cognitive and motor skills.

Because prematurity is so common for the majority of higher order multiples, it's important to recognize the potential consequences and be prepared for any eventuality. It's estimated that in 40 percent of supertwin births, at least one of the babies will suffer permanent physical or neurological damage due to complications. The risk can't be underestimated. The chapters in this book pertaining to preterm labor and premature babies will provide you with further information on the topic, as well as guidelines for improving the odds of a favorable outcome.

ALERT!

A normal singleton gestation is forty weeks. According to Mothers of Supertwins (M.O.S.T.), the average gestational age for triplets is 33.4 weeks. For quadruplets, it is 31 weeks. And for quintuplets, it is only 28.6 weeks.

Amid all the risks and complications, parents of higher order multiples should have optimistic hope. Advances in medical technology improve the odds for at-risk babies with every passing day. New drugs and treatments allow mothers to sustain their pregnancies longer, and neonatal care gives even extremely premature infants the opportunity to thrive.

Selective Reduction

One of the most controversial issues faced by parents of higher order multiples is the option of selective reduction. Many parents are horrified by the mere suggestion, while others firmly believe that it is the only way to ensure a healthy outcome.

Multifetal selective reduction is the practice of reducing a higher order multiple pregnancy, usually to a twin pregnancy, in order to minimize risk and maximize the potential viability of the remaining fetuses. During an outpatient procedure, a needle is inserted into the mother's uterus, either through the vagina or abdomen. Ultrasound guides the needle as it injects potassium chloride into one or more of the embryos. The chemical halts the embryo's development and the embryo is eventually reabsorbed by the body.

When It's Warranted

Medically, selective reduction is an accepted method of improving the odds. Despite the successful delivery of septuplets to the McCaughey family, many incidences of extreme multiple pregnancy result in the loss of some or all of the babies.

The procedure is usually recommended only in incidences of quadruplets or higher and is generally performed toward the end of the first trimester. That doesn't give parents a great deal of time to consider their options. They may feel pressured by the dire predictions of their doctors or conversely by their own religious or moral convictions. It is a tremendously agonizing decision, with no clear answer.

FACT

The facts show that every additional baby puts the entire pregnancy at risk. It's estimated that 70 percent of quadruplets will survive, and 50 percent of the survivors will suffer disabilities or impairment. But twins are given a much higher survival rate: 98 percent with only a 5 percent chance of suffering permanent impairment.

Making a Difficult Decision

If you are faced with making a decision regarding selective reduction, it's imperative that you receive qualified advice from a variety of sources. In most cases, parents are put into this position after undergoing extensive fertility enhancements to get pregnant in the first place, so most likely you will already have a good relationship with at least one professional in this area. Ask your reproductive specialist for objective statistical information regarding the potential outcomes for your pregnancy. In addition, consult a qualified perinatologist or other specialist in higher order multiple pregnancy. They may offer a different assessment of your pregnancy's potential.

Once you have compiled a balanced view of your options and the medical risks and benefits involved with each, you'll have to confront the emotional aspects of your situation. Because it is such a controversial issue, you may find it difficult to discuss with friends or family members, especially if they have strong opinions on the subject. Choose your confidantes carefully. It may be helpful to seek guidance from a trusted religious adviser who can help you reconcile your beliefs with your choices. Perhaps your most valuable resource at this difficult time is the support of families who have faced a similar choice. Networking with other parents will provide an opportunity for you to discuss the outcome of their choice, whether they decided for or against selective reduction.

There are several organizations that can provide support for parents facing this choice, including national groups such as M.O.S.T. Online or the Triplet Connection, as well as local chapters of multiples clubs. You'll find contact information for these and other organizations in Appendix A.

Preparing for Supertwins

It's not uncommon for families to have three, four, or five children. However, having them all at once is a completely different scenario! As you read through this book to prepare yourself for the birth of multiples, there are several things that you should keep in mind as a parent (or parent-to-be) of supertwins.

First of all, once the babies arrive, you'll be immediately outnumbered. Where parents of twins can divide their time equally between two babies, you'll always have someone waiting in the wings for your attention. In this type of situation, it is essential that you establish routines to ensure that everyone's needs are met.

Secondly, every additional baby represents an increase. Everything is "more." You'll need more help, have to buy more supplies, and require more medical monitoring. At the same time, your babies will likely have less time in your womb, so it's vital that you make the most of your pregnancy. You'll have to eat more—and gain more weight—than a mom of a singleton, or even twins. You'll need to get more rest and spend more time off your feet.

Finally, even though there are more demands, the rewards also increase exponentially. Your children will enjoy the spotlight of their special status as supertwins. They will share a unique bond with their same-age siblings. Your family will include a ready-made playgroup, and they will never be without companionship. And as parents, you can look forward to three times the smiles, four times the giggles, or five times as many hugs!

Chapter 4

The First Trimester

So you're pregnant! You may or may not even know that you're having multiples during the first twelve weeks of your pregnancy, but it is definitely a time of discovery, surprising physical changes, and emotional upheaval. If you've been pregnant before, you may think you know what to expect, but there are some unexpected differences when you're pregnant with more than one.

Signs and Symptoms of Multiples

Some mothers are fully aware that they are pregnant with two or more babies from the very beginning of their pregnancy. They may have strong and accurate powers of intuition or, more likely, they are under the supervision of a reproductive specialist who is monitoring every step of the conception process. However, most women who spontaneously conceive twins, triplets, or more won't begin to suspect anything out of the ordinary until their pregnancy progresses.

FACT

Multiples manifest their presence in several ways, but no one symptom distinguishes itself as a clear indicator. Some mothers of multiples report a strong suspicion based on one factor or combination of signals, while others experience absolutely nothing out of the ordinary.

Suspicious Signs

Any of the following indicators may come up in the first trimester. If you experience them to an unusually extreme degree, it may be a sign that you are carrying multiples.

- **Weight gain:** A singleton mother gains, on average, five to seven pounds in the first trimester. Anything more could indicate multiples . . . or excessive junk food consumption!
- **Abdomen size:** With multiple babies in her womb, a pregnant woman tends to outgrow her regular clothing and require maternity gear sooner. Although it is difficult to estimate fundal size (the size of the uterus) in early pregnancy, sometimes an increase is evident, indicating multiple babies.
- **Fatigue:** Excessive fatigue is one of the most commonly reported complaints of mothers of multiples in the early stages of pregnancy. With their bodies busy taking care of the babies, there is little energy left over for carrying out their daily routines.

- **Fetal movement:** It's very unusual for a mother to experience fetal movement in the first trimester, yet there is some evidence to suggest that the sensation is more acute when there is more than one baby moving around.
- **Nausea:** Extra babies can intensify the symptoms of morning sickness, such as nausea and vomiting.

You may be aware of some or all of these indications, or none at all. Perhaps your doctor or midwife brought the symptoms to your attention during a routine exam. However, they are also all normal consequences of pregnancy, which makes it quite difficult to tell whether they are truly a sign of multiples.

A Certain Something

In addition to physical symptoms, many mothers of multiples report an unexplainable hunch or vague suspicion early in pregnancy. Often it's triggered by unusual circumstances that bring multiples to the forefront of their attention. Perhaps they dream about having twins, or find themselves running across several sets of multiples in a public place. Or they may encounter mysterious phenomena that occur in sets of twos or threes. One expectant mother of twins discovered that the eggs she'd bought for holiday baking all contained double yolks; two days later an ultrasound revealed that she was having twins!

Hearing Heartbeats

You might assume that multiple babies would be easily identified by listening for multiple heartbeats. Unfortunately, that is not an effective practice in early pregnancy. Distinct heartbeat sounds are usually only detected toward the end of the first trimester, about week twelve. Even then, what sounds like an additional baby might actually be an echo of the mother's own beating heart. In other situations, multiple babies that are positioned fairly close together in the womb may have indistinguishable rhythms that are misinterpreted as a single heartbeat.

The phenomenon of one audible heartbeat is particularly common with monochorionic monozygotics (see Chapter 2). Not only do they have similar heart rhythms, but they tend to settle close to each other because they are contained in the same sac.

HCG Screening and Multiples

One of the earliest ways to detect the possibility of multiples is by monitoring the level of human chorionic gonadotropin (or HCG) in the mother's body. HCG is a hormone secreted by the fertilized egg(s). It regulates the production of other hormones, such as progesterone and estrogen, until the placenta develops and assumes that role.

HCG is the substance detected by common over-the-counter pregnancy tests to determine if a woman is pregnant or not. These tests measure the amount of HCG in a urine sample to determine whether there is enough of the hormone to indicate pregnancy.

But HCG monitoring of a blood sample provides a more comprehensive picture of the woman's status. It not only indicates whether an egg is fertilized, but can be used to determine whether the fertilized egg, implanted in the uterus, is developing into an embryo. An HCG blood test can also suggest the presence of more than one embryo.

Not every woman is a candidate for HCG monitoring. Many women never have their levels evaluated beyond a urine test to confirm pregnancy. However, some doctors do recommend testing, particularly in situations where there has been conception assistance or a history of miscarriage.

A single HCG measurement doesn't tell the story. Rather, samples are taken every few days during the early weeks of pregnancy and compared. With each passing day, increasing amounts of the hormone are detectable in the pregnant mother's system. HCG production peaks toward the end of the first trimester, so it is generally monitored only in the first few weeks of pregnancy.

HCG Levels in Single and Twin Pregnancy

Days from LMP*	HCG Range** for Singleton Pregnancy	HCG Range for Multiple Pregnancy
28	9.4–120	9.5–120
33	300–600	200–1,800
36	1,200–1,800	2,400–36,000
40	2,400–4,800	8,700–108,000
45	12,000–60,000	72,000–180,000
70	96,000–144,000	348,000–480,000

*LMP is the date of the start of the last menstrual period.
**HCG is measured in mIU/mL

As the chart illustrates, HCG measurements are quite inflated when a multiple pregnancy is present. However, they are not considered a completely reliable indicator of twins or more. In most cases, a high HCG reading will only prompt further investigation.

Confirming That There Is More Than One

The only way to authenticate a multiple pregnancy in the first trimester is with visual confirmation via ultrasound. Other indications and testing may arouse suspicion or contribute evidence, but you won't know anything for sure until you and your doctor peek inside through the magic of ultrasound technology.

Your caregiver may suspect multiples for several reasons. In addition to the symptoms and HCG indicators mentioned earlier, predisposition factors such as your age, a previous multiple pregnancy, history of twinning on your mother's side, or fertility treatment should always be considered valid reasons to screen for multiples early in the pregnancy.

Using Ultrasound

Some doctors routinely perform an ultrasound on their patients during their initial office visit, about a month into the pregnancy. Others wait until the second trimester, when a more comprehensive exam can be done to detect a wider range of issues. The American College of Obstetricians and Gynecologists is wary of routine ultrasound use in healthy pregnancy; however, diagnosing and monitoring multiple pregnancy is considered acceptable and is a recommended use of the technology.

If multiples are suspected, a brief ultrasound scan can help determine the proper course of action to ensure the healthiest possible outcome for mother and babies. Early detection of multiples is the best option for families, giving them more time to prepare physically and psychologically. Ultrasound technology can be successfully used to diagnose a multiple pregnancy as early as four weeks, but is generally used about halfway through the first trimester when individual heartbeats are distinguishable.

FACT

Advances in ultrasound technology mean that very few multiples make a surprise appearance during delivery. As recently as 1970, nearly half of twins, triplets, and other multiples went undetected, but in recent times, less than 10 percent remain undiagnosed.

Types of Ultrasound

Two types of ultrasound are used routinely in pregnancy: vaginal and abdominal. Generally, abdominal ultrasound is utilized later in pregnancy, while vaginal scans (also called transvaginal sonography or TVS) provide the most reliable information in the first trimester. A probe inserted into the vagina sends out high-frequency sound waves. As the waves bounce off the inner contours of the body, they are transmitted as electrical signals to a computer, which processes the results and displays a view of the womb on the screen.

Your doctor or radiologist will interpret the images to identify the cervix, uterus, and any embryonic or placental development. To parents, the images may appear as blobs or shadows, but the trained eye can clearly identify the number of embryos and their developing circulatory system, and can even pinpoint gestational age.

Just keep in mind that early ultrasound detection is not 100 percent accurate. Sometimes one embryo is shadowed behind another, and not visible using a two-dimensional scan. Ultrasound also can produce false evidence of multiple embryos if an empty sac is misinterpreted as a viable embryo.

Physical Changes

The first twelve weeks of a pregnancy are a very busy time, physically, for a mother of multiples. While your mind may be slow to adjust to the concept of having twins, triplets, or more, your body wastes no time in preparing to accommodate their needs in the womb. There are many different ways that you will experience the effects of the marvelous miracles growing inside you. In many aspects, the early pregnancy experience for mothers of multiples is very similar to a singleton situation. Some of the symptoms may be exaggerated, but they are generally of the same nature.

Changes in Your Digestive System

The impact on your digestive system is one of the most acute—and uncomfortable—side effects of pregnancy. Fluctuating hormones decrease the muscle tone of your stomach and intestines and slow down your ability to move food through the digestive tract. At the same time, your digestive organs are being crowded by your expanding uterus. The result? Heartburn, indigestion, nausea, vomiting, constipation, or a combination of all of the above!

Although it's called "morning sickness," this unpleasant stomach distress can occur at any hour of the day or night. Just as your appetite increases, your ability to process the food decreases. Everything may smell and taste different. You may crave foods that you didn't care for previously, while your stomach turns at the mere thought of old favorites. Believe it or not, morning sickness may actually be your body's way of protecting your unborn babies.

Some researchers believe that the nausea and vomiting are a way of ridding your body of potentially toxic chemicals and protecting the fetuses from harmful food-borne bacteria.

Every woman copes with morning sickness differently. What works as a solution for one pregnant woman may make symptoms worse in another. Trial and error will help you find the best remedy for your situation. Take heart; it's a temporary condition of pregnancy, and your symptoms will likely be alleviated by the second trimester.

Here are some common recommendations for relieving morning sickness:

- Graze. Small, frequent meals and regular snacks keep your stomach happy.
- Avoid greasy or fatty foods. They take longer to digest and stay in your stomach longer.
- Stay away from spicy fare. It can aggravate symptoms by irritating your stomach tissue.
- Have someone else prepare the food. Cooking odors may trigger nausea.
- Nibble on bland snacks that are high in carbohydrates and protein, such as whole grain crackers, low-fat yogurt, or nuts.
- Wear a nausea-controlling acupressure band, such as those sold to combat seasickness.
- Talk to your doctor about homeopathic remedies such as ginger or vitamin B_6 supplements.
- Don't rush out of bed in the morning. Give yourself time to relax and your stomach will too.

Morning sickness can be harmful if the vomiting becomes severe or excessive enough to result in dehydration. The condition, called hyperemesis gravidarum, occurs in about 5 percent of multiple pregnancies and requires medical treatment. Let your doctor know if you are unable to keep down any food or fluids over a twenty-four hour period.

Changes in Your Circulatory System

Your circulatory system will also experience major changes during pregnancy. Blood flows to and from the placenta(s) to deliver oxygenated blood and extract unoxygenated blood from the babies. There is a drastic increase in the amount of blood (blood volume) that your body has to circulate. Each additional baby increases the volume by about 10 percent.

You'll notice the impact of the increased blood volume in many different parts of your body. Swollen blood vessels in your nose and sinuses may cause stuffiness or even nosebleeds. Your gums may bleed when you brush or floss your teeth. Some women's heart rate becomes elevated.

That extra radiance known as "pregnancy glow" isn't simply a symptom of happiness at having multiples. It's caused by an increase in blood flowing close to the skin's surface. Enjoy the glow, but also be careful. Your skin may react more sensitively to the sun or skin-care products.

Your breasts may become swollen and sensitive. The nipples and areolae may darken and you might notice prominent blue veins, especially if your skin is particularly fair. Many women find that their bras are one of the first things they outgrow during pregnancy. Some mothers of multiples gain two or three cup sizes by the end of their pregnancy.

The pressure of the extra blood flow causes your veins to dilate. This phenomenon is the cause of varicose veins, one of the unfortunate effects of pregnancy that doesn't disappear after delivery. Another particularly unpleasant consequence is the development of hemorrhoids, which occurs when the veins around the rectum become enlarged and protruding. The majority of mothers of multiples have to contend with the resulting itching and discomfort throughout their pregnancy.

Drinking lots and lots of fluids, particularly water, helps your body accommodate the production of all that extra blood. You'll also benefit by upping your iron intake. You might notice that you're craving iron-rich foods such as red meat or leafy green vegetables. It's a good idea to discuss your iron intake requirements with your doctor, who might recommend supplements.

Weight Changes

In a normal singleton pregnancy, weight gain is minimal in the first trimester, usually less than five pounds. However, some would say that when you're carrying multiples, an earlier weight gain produces healthier babies, based on the assumption that twins and especially higher order multiples have a shorter gestational period. Unlike a singleton pregnancy, where most weight is accumulated in the later months, weight gain may be accelerated in the earlier months with multiples.

At the same time, excessive weight gain can produce its own set of problems, during pregnancy and beyond. Gestational diabetes, high blood pressure, and even postmenopausal breast cancer have been linked to unhealthy weight accumulation during pregnancy. In order to strike the right balance and achieve a healthy weight gain for both yourself and your babies, you need to be more aware of your weight fluctuations, beginning with the first trimester.

Weight gained in the first trimester is the hardest to get rid of postpartum, since it is composed mainly of fat stores. It is not until the second trimester that the combined weight of the babies and placentas are reflected in your weight total.

By the end of the first trimester, you will likely see the scale inch upward, especially after the tenth week. Some of the increase, about two pounds, can be attributed to the extra blood volume and retained fluid. The rest is primarily accumulated body fat. Some women, depending on the severity of their morning sickness or the shape they were in pre-pregnancy, actually lose weight. Your initial prenatal visit with your doctor or midwife is an excellent opportunity to discuss the issue. At that time, your caregiver should assess your weight goals based on your individual situation.

Other Early Effects

Some of the early effects of pregnancy are difficult to distinguish from your body's normal functions. But when there's more than one baby in the womb, these manifestations of impending maternity may be experienced more intensely. They are often a clue that there's something different about this pregnancy.

Fatigue

The one symptom most commonly experienced by expectant mothers of multiples appears to be fatigue. From occasional drowsiness to overwhelming exhaustion, nearly every pregnant woman feels her body's call to slow down and rest. It's not hard to imagine why. Before pregnancy, your body kept itself pretty busy taking care of your own needs. Now it has to attend to the demands of two, three, or even more additional beings. With the busy baby-building boom going on, there's not much energy left over for mom!

It's important to listen to your body's cues and give it the rest it requires. Take naps, go to bed earlier in the evening, and sleep late when possible. Fatigue is generally temporary, and most overwhelming during the first trimester. There is really no remedy for it, except to give in and rest.

ALERT!

Because the first trimester is such a crucial time in your babies' development, it's important that you do your best to take care of your body. Tobacco use, alcohol, exposure to toxic substances, and even stress can contribute to defects and disabilities and should be avoided.

Spotting or Bleeding

It's normal to have some spotting or bleeding during the first trimester, but that doesn't mean that it's not frightening. The appearance of blood can make an already emotional pregnant woman frantic with worry. The most common type of bleeding during the first trimester of pregnancy is sometimes called implantation bleeding. It coincides with the timing of the first missed period and is often misinterpreted as the onset of menstruation. Instead, it is merely a result of the fertilized eggs burrowing into the soft lining of the uterus. It is usually lighter than a menstrual period and should only last a day or so.

Bleeding or spotting can also occur for a variety of other reasons in the first trimester and does not necessarily indicate an impending miscarriage. The majority of women who experience bleeding go on to have a healthy pregnancy. You should, however, notify your doctor or midwife, especially if the blood is bright red or accompanied by cramping, pain, or fever.

Your Emotional State

There is nothing quite as shocking as the surprising revelation that you are carrying multiples. Whether you find out immediately after an assisted conception, or late into your pregnancy, the discovery that you are carrying two, three, or more babies pushes your pregnancy into a new dynamic. Suddenly you are labeled a "high-risk pregnancy." Immediately there are more worries. Along with a new level of excitement, the questions loom. What will go wrong? How will we cope? Can we afford this?

Your fluctuating hormones only serve to heighten the emotion of the moment. You may find yourself hysterically laughing at your unbelievable fortune one minute, then sobbing with distress the next. Mood swings are a normal consequence of pregnancy. The surging hormones affect the neurotransmitters in your brain that control your feelings; the sensation often peaks in the last half of the first trimester.

Talking to other families with multiples is extremely reassuring during your pregnancy. Appendix A of this book contains several resources for finding support, locally or online. As you come in contact with parents in similar situations, you'll see that life with twins, triplets, or more is truly a joyful experience, despite the challenges.

Don't fret if you feel overwhelmed or out of control. You still have several months to prepare for your new arrivals, and you'll be able to put that time to good use. Educating yourself about multiple birth—by reading this book, for example—is an excellent way to get a handle on your situation. As you learn more, you'll feel better equipped to handle the adventures ahead.

The Babies' Development in the First Trimester

Your babies have been very busy since their conception. They've evolved from a sperm and an egg into a zygote, traveled down the fallopian tubes, implanted in the uterus to become an embryo, and established a placenta. At the end of the first trimester, they officially graduate from embryos to fetuses, as they will be known for the duration of the pregnancy.

Setting up shop in your womb, they've developed within a cushioning fluid-filled sac called the amnion, where they lie protected by a second membrane called the chorion. Depending on their zygosity and exactly how the development of the zygotes began (see Chapter 2), two co-multiples may be sharing the space.

As early as four weeks post-conception, the embryos have established the foundation for many of their major organs. In each embryo a tiny heart beats. A brain and a primitive central nervous system have formed. By eight weeks, the skeletal system forms a network of bones and many organ systems begin to function. At the end of the first trimester, the babies will be about the size of a travel tube of toothpaste and weigh about an ounce apiece.

Chapter 5

The Middle Trimester

Welcome to the second trimester. After getting acquainted with pregnancy in the first trimester, you'll have a chance to settle in during the next few months. As you grow accustomed to the idea of having multiples—and grow physically!—you are likely to experience a period of relief and rejuvenation. The nausea and exhaustion of the first trimester often give way to a period of enhanced energy and vitality.

Ultrasounds and Tests

Throughout the second trimester, you and your babies will go through several tests and assessments. Some are prompted by the extra risks inherent in a multiple pregnancy, requiring more intensive monitoring than a singleton pregnancy. Others are routine assessments that are recommended for all pregnancies. It's important to know what each test is measuring, and how it will be performed.

Ultrasound

You may have already had an ultrasound or sonogram during the first trimester. In fact, it is often the method by which a multiple pregnancy is confirmed, and perhaps your own twins, triplets, or more were revealed in the shadowy blobs of an ultrasound image. In the second trimester of pregnancy, most physicians recommend a routine ultrasound, often called a structural ultrasound. Generally, this exam is scheduled at about twenty weeks. At this point in the pregnancy, the babies' anatomy is developed enough to be assessed, yet the babies are still small enough to be seen individually. Later in the pregnancy, as the womb becomes more crowded, their body parts may overlap and become more difficult to examine.

Your ultrasound may be performed by a trained sonographer, or by your obstetrician or perinatologist. Sometimes a Level II ultrasound is recommended for multiple pregnancies. This is simply a more detailed assessment. The same equipment is utilized but it is generally performed by a maternal-fetal specialist at a hospital rather than in your doctor's or midwife's office. It will likely take an hour or two, where a regular ultrasound lasts about thirty minutes.

Either way, the procedure provides much useful information. It helps to ascertain that the babies are developing on schedule, confirms their due date, and rules out potential problems such as Down syndrome, spina bifida, and hydrocephaly. Often other details are revealed, such as the babies' genders (if you want to make them known) and perhaps even their zygosity. During the procedure, your doctor will likely spend some time trying to identify and assess the membrane that separates the babies' sac. A discernible membrane may indicate that the babies are dichorionic, although it doesn't necessarily confirm that they are dizygotic. Even monozygotic (identical) twins can be dichorionic. A thin membrane might identify monochorionic twins while the lack of a membrane might be a clue that the babies are monoamnionic. (See Chapter 2 for more on zygosity.)

QUESTION?

Why is it important to detect the babies' gender in a multiple pregnancy?
Determining whether your babies are boys, girls, or one of each can help establish their zygosity. Only dizygotic (fraternal) multiples can be different sexes. Identifying that there are both male and female babies rules out monozygotic multiples and the associated complications, such as twin-to-twin transfusion syndrome and monoamniotic twin issues.

In addition, the doctor or sonographer will examine the placenta(s), assess the level of amniotic fluid for each baby, and measure the babies to estimate their weight. At twenty weeks, each multiple should weigh about one pound. In addition to getting a good look at the babies, a second trimester ultrasound is also a good time to check the length of your cervix. A long cervix is tightly closed, an encouraging sign that preterm labor is not imminent.

Ultrasound assessments can be a very enjoyable and reassuring test for expectant parents, offering them a peek at their developing babies. There are no known risks associated with ultrasound technology and it generates little discomfort for the mother, other than requiring her to lie flat during the procedure. You may have one ultrasound in the second trimester, but you are more likely to have several with a multiple pregnancy, as it is a simple, inexpensive, and relatively noninvasive diagnostic tool.

Technological advancements in ultrasound provide an even more detailed and defined picture of your womb. Doppler technology, familiar to many as a weather forecasting tool, makes it possible to monitor fetal blood flow and diagnose cardiac conditions. Three-dimensional (3-D) imaging allows you to view the womb in detail, while 4-D ultrasound incorporates movement in real time, providing a very lifelike look at the developing babies. Not only is it a heartwarming and exciting experience for parents, but it also creates the opportunity for more accurate evaluation and diagnosis of fetal conditions.

Your ultrasound technician may be able to print pictures of your ultrasound scan or even create a video for you to keep. Save them as a special souvenir of your pregnancy—your babies' first portraits!

Alpha-fetoprotein (AFP) Test

The Alpha-fetoprotein test is also commonly referred to as a triple screen test or multiple marker screening. It is normally offered in the second trimester, usually after the fifteenth week. It is intended as a screening for birth defects, but many women decline to take it because of the high rate of false positive results. A woman pregnant with multiples will produce an abnormal result, due to the increased levels of hormones produced by additional babies. In fact, many spontaneous twin pregnancies are identified in the second trimester after an AFP test returns a positive, or abnormal, result.

The test requires you to have blood drawn, which is sent to a lab to be analyzed. Three components are assessed: alpha-fetoprotein, a substance produced by the fetal liver; human chorionic gonadotropin (HCG), a pregnancy hormone; and unconjugated estriol (uE3), another hormone associated with pregnancy. A quadruple screen may also measure inhipin A, to detect Down syndrome.

Glucose Testing for Gestational Diabetes

Late in the second trimester, you will likely be screened for gestational diabetes. The test measures the amount of glucose in your blood to determine whether pregnancy hormones have affected the way that your body processes insulin. In most cases, the glucose level is assessed via a blood sample. Your doctor will provide you with a sweet, high-glucose beverage and instructions on when to drink it. About an hour later, blood will be drawn and sent to the lab. If your blood serum glucose level is high, you may be at risk for gestational diabetes. Usually a second round of more inten-sive testing, called an oral glucose tolerance test, is prescribed. You may be required to follow a special diet for a few days, or fast the night before. It can be a time-consuming test, since your blood will be drawn several times.

FACT

In a singleton pregnancy, gestational diabetes screening is usually performed early in the third trimester, but many doctors recommend earlier testing for moms of multiples. The risk of gestational diabetes is nearly doubled for moms expecting more than one baby.

Amniocentesis (Amnio)

Between the fourteenth and twentieth week of your pregnancy, you may be scheduled for an amniocentesis. During the process of amniocentesis, or amnio, your caregiver uses an ultrasound-guided needle to withdraw fluid from the babies' amniotic sac. Analysis of the fluid sample, which contains fetal cells, provides a wealth of information about the babies.

Amniocentesis may produce some cramping and you'll probably be advised to take it easy after the procedure. There are some inherent risks; the needle's invasion of the uterus can trigger infection, preterm labor, or even miscarriage. In a multiple pregnancy, in which each baby's amniotic sac must be sampled, the risks may be increased. Generally, this procedure is recommended for mothers over the age of thirty-five, or whose families have a history of chromosomal abnormalities or birth defects. It may also be warranted if there is an indication that you will deliver your babies prema-turely, as it can be an effective tool for assessing their lung maturity.

Chorionic Villus Sampling (CVS)

A newer alternative to amniocentesis is chorionic villus sampling (CVS). It is generally performed earlier in pregnancy, even as early as the first tri-mester. Chorionic villi are tiny tentacles of tissue projecting from the chorion that provide a sample of the babies' genetic material. A catheter is inserted through either the cervix or the abdominal wall to extract a sample of the villi.

E ALERT!

Although it is an extremely accurate tool for detecting genetic disorders, the risk of miscarriage after CVS is even 1 to 2 percent higher than with amniocentesis. It can be a challenging procedure when there are multiples, especially if they share a placenta. Your doctor will advise you as to the risks and benefits of undergoing such testing.

Your Body's Changes

Boy, is your body busy during the second trimester! By this time it is generally very difficult to conceal your pregnancy. The height of your fundus, the name for the top of your uterus, exceeds that of a singleton pregnancy by several inches. In fact, by the end of the second trimester, you may have the appearance of a full-term singleton pregnancy, causing you to attract concern for your "imminent" delivery.

What You're Feeling

The second trimester brings good news and bad news. Some of the problems that plagued you during the early weeks of pregnancy will start to dissipate, such as the nausea and queasiness of morning sickness and the extreme exhaustion. However, in their place, some new symptoms may make an appearance.

Your appetite may increase to ravenous proportions. Take advantage of your hunger to fill up on healthy foods, such as lean proteins, fresh fruit and vegetables, and whole grains. As your constant urge to urinate eases, you may find it easier to sleep through the night. However, you may be visited by frequent, vivid dreams.

One physical phenomenon that pregnant mothers of multiples are particularly prone to is round ligament pain, sharp pinching discomfort in the abdominal area. It occurs as the ligaments that support your uterus stretch to accommodate its rapid expansion. Sometimes it will happen when you move or stretch suddenly, or it can come out of the blue, even while you're at rest. Aside from the discomfort, it can be an alarming experience if you confuse the sensation with the onset of contractions. Round ligament pain usually eases after a moment, but if it recurs, be sure to discuss your symptoms with your doctor.

As you grow, your skin stretches to cover your expanding abdomen. Stretch marks may make an appearance on your breasts, belly, or hips. They indicate a separation of collagen, a substance that lends elasticity to skin. They may be pink or purplish, but will probably fade to a light silvery shadow after pregnancy. Stretch marks don't hurt, but they may feel tight or itchy. Lotions or oils can decrease the discomfort.

Some other common symptoms that you may experience during these middle months are

- Constipation
- Swelling (edema)
- Nasal stuffiness
- Bleeding gums
- Headaches

There is some good news. Many women attain a radiant appearance during this period of pregnancy. The extra circulation drives more blood to the hair follicles, skin surface, and nail beds. The result? Thick, lustrous hair; clear, luminous skin; and strong nails that grow faster than you can say "manicure." Enjoy the beauty effects of this special time!

Changes in Sexual Desire

After a few months of wanting sleep rather than sex, you may experience an awakening in the second trimester. Many moms, and appreciative dads, report an increase in sexual desire during this time. Sometimes extreme concern about preterm labor may prompt your caregiver to recommend abstinence, but unless you've been advised to restrict sexual activity, you can take advantage of your increased appetite. Most couples will enjoy a second honeymoon period before the advancing pregnancy literally gets in the way of sexual relations.

The Babies' Development

Your babies are having a busy season as well. Having developed into recognizable human form, they enter the second trimester with the appearance of newborns, only smaller. In the second trimester, they grow rapidly, from about twenty grams to nearly a pound in weight. By the end of the second trimester, they are each about eight inches in length.

At that size, they still have plenty of room to move around in the womb environment, and you are likely to experience their gymnastics routines with increasing frequency and intensity. Most mothers of multiples detect the sensation of fetal movement, called *quickening*, earlier than moms of singletons; however, if you've never been pregnant before, it's easy to mistake the feeling for gastrointestinal bubbles.

Most expectant mothers experience quickening by the twentieth week of pregnancy, but it's not uncommon for moms of multiples to discern the feeling as early as twelve weeks.

As the second trimester passes, the babies will become more and more active. They'll establish rhythms of activity and rest according to your routines, although often in contradiction to your schedule. For example, during the times of day when you're most active, your body movements lull them into tranquility, yet you'll find them wide awake and most active when you're still.

Weight Gain

Most women are particularly concerned with how their pregnancy will impact their body. Gaining weight is a given during pregnancy, and as you might expect, the amount of weight increases in a multiple pregnancy. In a singleton pregnancy, the average woman gains between twenty-five and thirty pounds during her pregnancy. Only a third of that is fat and maternal tissue; the rest is a combination of the baby, placenta, amniotic fluid, and increased blood volume. When you double or triple the number of babies, you can expect the amount to increase proportionately.

What to Gain

The amount of weight that you gain during your multiple pregnancy is dependent on a number of factors. Your pre-pregnancy size is one determinant. If you are overweight before becoming pregnant you'll need to gain less than if you were underweight. Your doctor can advise you as to the optimal amount for your individual situation, but a general guideline is thirty-five to forty-five pounds for twins, up to fifty-five pounds for triplets, and ten additional pounds per baby for higher order multiples.

Recommended Weight Gain in Multiple Pregnancy (in pounds)

Multiples	First Trimester	Second Trimester	Third Trimester	Total
Twin Pregnancy	5–10	15–20	10–20	35–45
Triplet Pregnancy	5–10	20–30	20–25	45–60
Quadruplet Pregnancy	10–15	25–35	20–25	50–75
Quintuplets Plus	10–20	25–35	25–30	65–100

When to Gain

The timetable of your weight gain is every bit as important as the amount. In a multiple pregnancy it is particularly important to gain weight early, prior to the third trimester. Because multiple pregnancies are often cut short due to preterm delivery, more weight has to be gained in a shorter amount of time. Gaining steadily throughout the first and second trimesters helps you establish extra stores of fat and nutrients. The babies will rely on those stockpiled deposits in later pregnancy when their nutritional demands are greater.

The amount of weight you gain in the first half of your pregnancy has a significant impact on your babies' development in the second half. The pounds you accumulate now will help sustain them later.

In the second trimester, you should aim to gain one to one-and-a-half pounds per week, depending on your situation and the number of babies that you're carrying. In the first trimester, decreased appetite due to the effects of morning sickness may have inhibited your weight accumulation. Take advantage of your ravenous appetite in mid-pregnancy to feed yourself—and your babies—plenty of nutritious food.

Think Positive

For many women, weight gain carries complex psychological and emotional baggage. The idea of gaining nearly fifty pounds or more can be frightening and staggering. Try to keep it in perspective. Gaining the weight is a good thing; it's a sign of healthy development for your babies. Remember, too, that a good percentage of your weight gain will be lost at delivery. Finally, keep in mind that you're not just adding pounds; you're adding two or more new members to your family. In comparison, you'd likely accumulate more weight if you had serial singleton pregnancies.

Maternity Clothes

It's time to go shopping! By the second trimester, you'll have outgrown your pre-pregnancy outfits and will require maternity clothing. Before you spend a bundle on new attire, you'll want to consider the big picture, which is growing bigger every week! While you should have no problem fitting into standard maternity styles during this middle trimester, you may need to update your wardrobe every few weeks to accommodate your escalating girth.

The most important factor in choosing clothing is comfort. Choose soft, flexible fabrics with a bit of stretch to accommodate your girth. Recent fashion trends have produced new styles of maternity clothing that sit below the belly, instead of stretching across it, and many women find this a more comfortable option. It's also more practical for moms of multiples, whose bellies exceed the measurements of the average pregnancy.

Consider your lifestyle and activities when selecting clothes. Many of your pre-pregnancy routines will be altered in the months ahead; you may have a reduced work or social schedule and won't require as many special occasion outfits as you did previously. A few pairs of comfortable pants in basic colors are a good foundation. Mix and match with a variety of tops and blouses to extend your options. Remember that your bustline may expand as your pregnancy progresses, so consider tops with roomy armholes and a generous fit across the bust. When buying skirts or dresses, choose hemlines that fall below the knee. As your belly grows, it will pull up the fabric of your skirts, risking an overexposure of your thighs!

FACT

Generally, manufacturers advise women to buy maternity clothing according to their pre-pregnancy size. However, mothers of twins or multiples may wish to size up. Buy one or two sizes bigger in anticipation of your expansion in the months ahead.

Maternity clothing can be a big expense in pregnancy. If you have any opportunity to borrow outfits, take advantage of that! Some local clubs for parents of twins organize maternity clothing swaps or sales. Consignment shops are another good option for bargains.

Special Considerations for Higher Order Multiples

If you are expecting triplets or more, the second trimester is a special time. The likelihood of restricted activity, bed rest, hospitalization, or early delivery looms large in the third trimester, so it's especially important for you to utilize your time in these middle months wisely.

While you're feeling up to it, plan to do your shopping to stock up on supplies and get your home ready for the new arrivals. Schedule time together with your spouse or with your older children. The changes facing your family in the months ahead will prevent you from enjoying quiet time for quite a while. But don't overdo it. You don't want to raise your risk of complications by pushing yourself too hard.

Chapter 6

The Final Trimester

You're getting close! The final trimester with multiples may be a few weeks shorter than a singleton pregnancy, but it can feel like an eternity to a pregnant mother who is growing increasingly uncomfortable. But it's also a time of great joy and anticipation, and of finalizing some important decisions and preparation.

Staying Comfortable

There's no doubt about it, the last few months of a multiple pregnancy can get uncomfortable. For one thing, you've expanded to accommodate two or more growing babies! You may feel gigantic, and realize that you're only growing larger. Despite your overall lack of energy and a stern admonition from your doctor to rest as much as possible, your increased girth may make it impossible to relax comfortably. Meanwhile, as they grow, the babies are putting increasing pressure on your muscles, ribs, lungs, stomach, and bladder. As the time to deliver draws near, your emotional discomfort may increase as well. Fears about your babies' safe entry into this world and your future as a family may seem more relevant as the time of their arrival gets closer.

Life in the third trimester doesn't have to be miserable, however. Keep your situation in perspective; it's temporary, after all. Despite the physical discomfort they cause inside of you, your babies are much better off in your womb than born prematurely. This is a time for frequent positive reinforcement and support; remind yourself that things could be much worse and adopt an attitude of gratitude for each extra day of nurturing that you can give your babies.

Dressing for Success

You may find that you've outgrown your maternity wardrobe. Aside from a tent, your options for clothing are limited. Even the largest sizes of maternity wear may not cover your expanded midsection. Many mothers find that the best option for late pregnancy is to skip the maternity store and invest in a couple of plus-size outfits. Designed to accommodate larger women, they should fit comfortably over your belly. You don't need much to carry you through these last few months; a few T-shirts and elastic-waist pants will do. You may have to sacrifice fashion for a while, but you can look forward to returning to style once the babies are born.

It's not just clothing that doesn't seem to fit right in the last few months. You may have problems getting your shoes on your feet, and not just because your belly is in the way. Pregnancy hormones soften up the ligaments in your body, and your feet actually expand. You may find that yours have increased a size or two, and your shoes don't fit anymore. Since you may spend some portion of the third trimester off your feet, you don't need to invest a lot of money in new shoes. Comfort is the utmost priority, and so is convenience. Unless you want to get help with lacing and tying, slip-on shoes are the best option for the latter stage of pregnancy.

ALERT!

Even if you lose weight after you deliver, your feet may not ever return to their old shoe size. A pregnancy hormone called relaxin softens up joints and ligaments, including those in feet. Sometimes this causes feet to spread out and widen, and they don't always return to their pre-pregnancy shape.

If you are plagued by backache and muscle discomfort, you may want to invest in an undergarment that supports the weight of your expanding belly. It helps take the pressure off of your back and can provide a great deal of relief. You'll find such products available at maternity and baby stores, and the cost may be covered by your insurance plan. Buy a product intended for late pregnancy, even if you plan to start wearing it before the third trimester. As a mother of multiples, you'll need the extra support earlier in your pregnancy.

A good bra will also provide comfort. As your breasts prepare for nursing, they are likely changing shape and size, and your pre-pregnancy bras won't fit the bill, so to speak. If you haven't already, invest in several good-quality maternity bras. If you're planning to breastfeed, you can even consider starting to wear nursing bras. They'll do double duty, providing extra support for the last few months of your pregnancy, and easy access to your breasts once the babies arrive.

Working It Out

If she hasn't already, your doctor may advise you to stop working during the last portion of your pregnancy. Any job that requires a lot of standing, strenuous physical activity, or long hours is probably not a good way to spend the last weeks before the babies are born. However, some mothers are able to continue at their jobs until shortly before they deliver. Discuss the risks and benefits with your medical provider if you are having twins and your job allows you to be relatively sedate and comfortable while you work. Mothers of higher order multiples will likely have less opportunity to stay on the job.

If you do continue to work, take it easy. Stay off your feet as much as possible. Take frequent breaks and drink plenty of water throughout your workday. If your job involves repetitive hand motion, such as typing or filing nails, carpal tunnel syndrome may make the activity uncomfortable. It's made worse during pregnancy when increased blood volume through arteries and veins compresses the nerves in the hands and wrist, resulting in tingling, numbness, or pain.

The symptoms of carpal tunnel syndrome can be alleviated by wearing a splint or restricting activity, but ultimately the only thing that will make it go away is delivery of the babies.

On the Go

As it gets closer to the time when your babies will arrive, your list of "to-do's" gets longer and longer. Unfortunately, you may find that you're less productive in the last trimester. You may experience difficulty getting in and out of a car; you may even need to restrict your driving if your shape prevents you from sitting safely behind the wheel. This is a great time to take advantage of Internet services and do your shopping from the comfort of home.

As relaxing as it may sound, this is not the time to plan a vacation getaway. While mothers of singletons are considered safe for air travel up to week thirty-six, that's not the case with mothers of multiples, who are at increased risk for preterm labor. Many airlines have policies denying travel to women in the last month of their pregnancy; with twins or more, you'll look like you're near your due date even if you're months away. If your doctor does give you permission to travel by air (which is unlikely in the third trimester), you will need a letter indicating that you can safely fly in order to board the aircraft.

At Home

You may feel inclined to "nest" as your due date gets closer, making your home clean and ready for the babies. Leave the heavy-duty work to someone else, however. Activities that require heavy lifting, pushing, or climbing are simply too risky. Slaving over a hot stove isn't recommended either, although short bouts of standing in the kitchen may be acceptable. If your doctor approves, use that nesting energy to make and freeze casseroles to eat later; you'll likely have less time to prepare meals when you're busy feeding the babies.

When Will You Deliver?

As you reach the third trimester, the birth of your babies may seem imminent. With so much attention focused on the risks of preterm labor, you may be anticipating an early arrival. (Chapter 14 deals with the risks and signs of preterm labor in detail.) Even though you've made it past the critical point for survival, your babies will benefit by spending the majority of the third trimester in your womb, rather than in the hospital.

For many mothers of multiples, the last trimester is cut short. About half of twins, and the majority of higher order multiples, are born at least a month early. It's important to remain aware of the signs of preterm labor. You'll be scheduled for more frequent visits with your health-care provider so that he can assess any signs of impending labor, as well as the condition of your babies.

Testing for Preterm Labor

Fetal fibronectin testing allows doctors to predict whether preterm labor is imminent, although it doesn't provide any guarantees unless the test provides a negative return. Fetal fibronectin (FFN) is a protein found in the membranes and fluid of the amniotic sac. If its presence is detected in the area of the mother's cervix or vagina between twenty-four and thirty-four weeks' gestation, it could indicate the onset of preterm labor, even when other symptoms aren't apparent. Your doctor or midwife may perform a fetal fibronectin test in the third trimester to assess your risk of early delivery.

A negative test can be reassuring; your chances of delivering preterm are less than 10 percent. A positive is less conclusive. The detection of fetal fibronectin doesn't necessarily mean that labor is imminent, but it will probably require you to be closely monitored.

Fetal Assessment

During the last trimester, you're likely to have ample opportunity to keep tabs on your babies. Fetal surveillance during the last trimester is accomplished with ultrasound and heart rate monitoring, with a variety of tests that determine the babies' condition. A nonstress test is a painless way for you to participate in assessing the babies. It's performed by your doctor, usually at about thirty weeks, although it can be used earlier in pregnancy to monitor the impact of contractions. Testing is done with transducers that measure each baby's heart rate, and an additional monitor to record any uterine contractions. You'll be asked to sit quietly or lie down and relax. Remember, it's called a *non*stress test, so don't be anxious! As the transducers monitor the babies' heart rates, you'll be asked to indicate your experience of fetal movement.

A nonstress test is one component of a biophysical profile, a test that gives an overall assessment of the babies' condition. It's usually recommended midway through the last trimester, beginning at about week thirty-two. It includes evaluations of each baby's heart rate activity, respiration, body movements, muscle tone, and amniotic fluid volume. It may also include an assessment of the placenta. The nonstress test provides information about the fetuses' heart rate activity, while the rest of the elements are measured via ultrasound. If one or more of the babies scores low on a biophysical profile, it may be cause for concern and may prompt consideration of an early delivery.

Overdue and Over It

Despite the focus on preventing preterm labor, not all multiples are born early. Half of twin pregnancies last longer than thirty-six weeks. You may find yourself in the final weeks of the third trimester feeling like there is no end in sight. It can be an uncomfortable time, full of relief that your babies are close to term, but with anxiety looming about labor and delivery.

There is medical evidence to suggest that postmature pregnancy poses risks for both the babies and their mother. The discomfort of late-term pregnancy and the strain on the mother's organs may prompt doctors to intervene if labor is not imminent. Some argue that thirty-eight weeks should be considered full term for twins and recommend delivery when a mother reaches that point. Other experts maintain that forty weeks is the standard milestone, whether there is one baby or more.

Because the risk of preterm birth is heightened for multiples, much attention is focused on delivering early, rather than late. However, a review of the National Organization of Mothers of Twins Clubs' database indicates that 13 percent of its membership didn't deliver before their due date.

Whether early or late, it's difficult to predict the exact date of your babies' arrival. Throughout the final trimester, your medical care providers will review the babies' status and your own health. Your body may go into labor on its own—ideally, close to term, but possibly earlier. Or your doctor may recommend an intervention to deliver the babies in an effort to optimize their health or your own well-being. You will have to work as a team with your medical advisor to determine the best possible course of action to ensure a healthy outcome.

Making a Birth Plan

A birth plan has become a standard practice for expectant mothers who want to maintain some level of control over their birth experience. It is a document that communicates your wishes and expectations to the medical professionals who will be participating in your care. It is not intended to be antagonistic or confrontational, and should respect both your concerns and the caregivers' expertise.

What's the Point?

Moms of multiples who prefer to retain some control over their birth experience may be frustrated by the increased level of medical intervention required when there are twins or more. A written birth plan is a good way to express your desires regarding the birth in a way that optimizes the medical staff's ability to accommodate you.

It's important to develop your birth plan in plenty of time before you actually give birth. Given the risk of preterm labor, that can be earlier rather than later in a multiple pregnancy. The first part of the third trimester is an excellent time to start developing it. You'll want to provide ample time to review your plan with the appropriate caregivers, including your obstetrician, perinatologist, midwife, doula, pediatrician, and neonatologist. Be willing to discuss any concerns they might have, and once you've finalized the plan, ask them to sign the document to indicate their approval of your requests. Ask that a copy be placed in your medical chart. In addition, bring several copies of the signed plan to the hospital with you, so that you can share them with any other staff members who are assigned to care for you or the babies.

Things to Include in Your Plan

Your plan should encompass any aspects of the birth process that you have strong feelings about. Include references to any options for labor, delivery, recovery, postpartum care, breastfeeding, circumcision, and newborn care. State the names of any people whom you want involved in your care, including your spouse/partner, coach, or doula. Be sure to specify your preferences for each baby by clear references to Baby A, Baby B, and so on.

ALERT!

While your birth plan should be comprehensive, keep it concise. Significant information will be overlooked if it's too wordy. Keep it short and simple, and you're more likely to have it implemented to your satisfaction.

Some important items to address in your birth plan are below.
During labor:

- ❏ Mobility (being able to walk around)
- ❏ Access to food and liquids
- ❏ Placement of IVs
- ❏ Atmosphere of the labor environment (control of lights, noise)
- ❏ Administration of pain medication
- ❏ Anesthesia preferences
- ❏ Nonmedical pain relief options
- ❏ Performance of vaginal exams
- ❏ Presence of support persons
- ❏ Limits on visitors, including observation by medical students

During delivery:

- ❏ Episiotomy options
- ❏ Ability to record the birth
- ❏ Pushing position
- ❏ Avoidance of unnecessary intervention
- ❏ Cutting of the umbilical cord, including a request for a partner to cut it

In the event of a c-section:

- ❏ Anesthesia preferences
- ❏ Catheterization preferences
- ❏ Presence of partner during procedure
- ❏ Ability to remain alert

Postpartum:

- ❏ Rooming-in preferences
- ❏ Feeding instructions
- ❏ Privacy requests, including private room preference

Issues specific to multiples:

❑ Attempts to turn second baby before delivery (external cephalic version)
❑ Ability to see and hold babies between deliveries
❑ Interactions with neonatology staff in the event your babies are admitted
❑ Requests for co-bedding

Ultimately, make your birth plan flexible and accommodating of emergencies and contingencies. Recognize that you and the medical professionals who treat you have the same goal: a safe delivery and healthy babies.

FACT

You can find more assistance with developing a birth plan in pregnancy books and online. A particularly good resource for multiple birth labor and delivery has been developed by Karen Kerkhoff Gromada and is available on her Web site (✎www.karengromada.com).

Preparing for Delivery

In most cases, giving birth to multiples will require a hospital visit. Although some mothers of multiples opt to deliver at home or at a birthing center, it is generally not recommended for the safety of all involved. Instead, a hospital equipped with a Level III NICU (neonatal intensive care unit) can provide optimal care for multiples in the event that they require extra care. The third trimester is a good time to begin preparing for your hospital visit.

What to Pack

Often the onset of labor comes unexpectedly. If you put off packing your bag and making arrangements, you may be caught unprepared. It's a good idea to start assembling the things that you need so that you're ready when the time comes.

If you're being hospitalized for preterm labor, you'll need additional comfort items and entertainment to help you pass the time. If you're headed for the hospital planning to deliver, you'll need to consider the babies' needs in addition to your own.

For labor you'll need:

❑ Comfortable nightgowns (not pajamas)
❑ Underwear (comfortable old pairs are best; they may get messy)
❑ Socks
❑ Watch or stopwatch
❑ Pain management tools (focal point picture, massage balls, music)
❑ Camera
❑ Journal and pen

For recovery you'll want to have:

❑ Sanitary pads (they'll also be provided by the hospital)
❑ Address book or a list of people to contact with the good news
❑ Bathrobe
❑ Slippers or socks
❑ Essential toiletries

ALERT!

Don't pack anything expensive or irreplaceable. Things disappear easily in the hospital. Since most hospital bedding is white, put colorful pillowcases on any pillows you bring from home, and they won't get mixed in with the hospital laundry.

For going home:

❑ Car seats
❑ Clothing for each baby (don't forget coverings for heads and feet!)
❑ Baby blankets
❑ An outfit for you to wear home (not pre-pregnancy size)

If you plan to nurse, consider packing:

❏ Nursing bra
❏ Nursing pads or breast shields

Coverage at Home

Depending on how you deliver, you can expect to be away from home for at least a night or two. If you have a c-section, it can be four nights or more. You'll need to arrange coverage of your responsibilities at home while you're away.

If you have other children, arrange to have someone come and stay with them in your home. It will be less disruptive for them to remain in familiar surroundings. Have a backup plan in case you have to make a hasty departure for the hospital and your original arrangements fall through.

Pets also need care while you're away. Have a neighbor or pet sitter stop by to feed and walk your animals as needed. Your pets need the extra attention during this time of transition for your family.

Get your pets accustomed to the scent of your new arrivals before you bring the babies home. Send home a blanket or piece of clothing that has been touching the babies' skin and allow your dog or cat to take a whiff.

You'll want to share the good news about your babies with everyone you know, but you may be unable to spend a lot of time spreading the word while you recover. Instead, record a greeting on your answering machine so that friends and family can call to get updates. Or, designate a contact person to provide information. You'll only have to make one phone call, and your helper can do the rest.

Choosing Names for Your Multiples

Selecting names for your children is one of the most important decisions you will make on their behalf. It can be a difficult decision, especially considering that you have yet to meet the little ones you're assigning this lifelong label to. With multiples, you not only have to consider the individual nomenclature, but you'll also want to think about how their names interact as a group.

Naming style is a source of controversy among the multiples community. Some families try to avoid names that rhyme, start with the same letter, or otherwise appear matched. They feel that it compromises their multiples' sense of individuality. Others enjoy choosing a corresponding combination that clearly indicates their children's status as multiples. Ultimately, it's a matter of personal preference. You will find, however, that there is an expectation that twins and multiples' names should be coordinated, and you may be met with a reaction of disappointment if you announce unrelated names.

To start the process, brainstorm a list of names that you and your partner like. You can turn to baby-naming books and Web sites for ideas. If you know the sex of your babies, you can focus exclusively on names that match their gender. Have some backups for the opposite sex, though, just in case there was a mistake!

Once you have a list of possibilities, consider how the names work in combination. Even if you want to avoid matching names, you will probably want to select names with similar styles or a sense of balance—for example, names that are all very feminine, monosyllabic, or of comparable meaning. Keep in mind any potential nicknames for each choice.

QUESTION?

How do we decide which baby receives which name?
That can be a tricky determination. In utero, most multiples are identified by the labels "Baby A," "Baby B," "Baby C," and so on. You might select names that start with those letters. Other families assign names based on birth order. The first baby to be delivered receives one name, and the second another.

Can't come up with anything? There's no rule that you have to choose names before the babies arrive. Brainstorming names can be a fun diversion during labor. Or, you may wait until you meet them to make a decision. Laying eyes on your precious newborns might provide the inspiration to make the perfect choice.

Baby Showers for Multiples

A baby shower is a wonderful celebration of impending birth, and having multiples gives you even more to celebrate! The third trimester is the traditional time to have a shower.

Usually a baby shower is hosted by friends, neighbors, or relatives of the expectant parents. Because of the special considerations of a multiple pregnancy, you should discuss your situation with your hosts. They should be happy to accommodate you; after all, they want the best for you and the babies! Share your concerns regarding your pregnancy and acknowledge that your condition may impact your ability to participate. Let them know any specific needs or wants regarding baby supplies and equipment.

But don't wait too long. A baby shower for twins should be scheduled early enough in the third trimester that the mother is still comfortable and active. The risks of preterm labor and the potential for enforced bed rest could preclude Mom from attending her own shower. If you're having triplets, quadruplets, or more, you'll probably be better able to participate fully in the celebration if it's held before thirty weeks.

On the other hand, it's perfectly acceptable to reschedule a shower for after the babies are born, even if you have to wait several weeks until they come home from the hospital. After all, the babies are the guests of honor, and it's only fair that they get to attend. In many ways, it's more practical, too. By that time, you'll have a better idea of what you need, and your guests can tailor their gift-giving appropriately. Be forewarned; you'll lose your status as the star of the show if you have to compete with the babies at your own party. They're sure to win the hearts and attention of everyone in attendance.

If a shower is scheduled for later in the third trimester, an expectant mother of multiples may be most comfortable if the shower is planned to take place in her own home—assuming that she does not have responsibility for party preparations such as cooking or cleaning. She should just settle into the couch and let the party take place around her.

FACT

Being hospitalized for preterm labor didn't stop actress Julia Roberts from having a baby shower during her twin pregnancy. In October 2004, friends and family simply changed the location of the party, setting up the celebration in the hospital so she could attend.

Baby showers are a nice way for parents of multiples to stock up on all the extra supplies they need for their additional babies. Don't hesitate to make your needs known to your guests; they are eager to provide a gift that is useful or meaningful. In addition to baby clothing, supplies, and equipment, group contributions toward expensive items, such as strollers, cribs, or high chairs, would be welcomed. Sometimes the best gifts aren't things at all, but rather contributions of time or service. Offers to babysit, run errands, deliver meals, or provide transportation are some of the most appreciated gifts.

A baby shower tradition that will be truly treasured for years to come is the signing of a guest book. Encourage guests to write greetings to the parents-to-be, as well as the babies-to-come. Experienced parents may want to include words of wisdom or advice for the couple as they begin their journey as parents of multiples.

Chapter 7

E Having a Healthy
Pregnancy

Having multiples puts extra demands on the mother's body. In order to ensure the vitality of both mom and babies, it's important to make health a priority. There are many steps you can take to preserve and even improve your overall health while you're pregnant with multiples. You know you should be eating right and getting enough sleep, but do you know exactly what that means? It's also important to be aware of the things you should avoid during pregnancy.

What Should I Eat?

With so many facets of a multiple pregnancy beyond your control, your diet is one way that you can directly contribute to your babies' healthy development—what you eat is passed along to the babies through the placenta. It's important not only to eat the right foods, but also to consume enough food to satisfy everyone's nutritional needs.

Plenty of Protein

Research has suggested that protein plays an important role in fetal development. The amino acids found in animal proteins, such as meats, milk, and eggs, are an important component in the creation of human cells. These essential acids cannot be produced by the body but are consumed through the food you eat.

ALERT!

Be careful, though—not all sources of protein are the same. Many sources of animal protein have the disadvantage of being high in fat. It's important to select lean sources of protein. You can also eat a combination of other plant sources of protein to provide the essential acids that your body needs. These include rice and beans, peanut butter, whole grains, and soy.

It's recommended that the average woman consume about 10 percent of her calories in protein, or about 50 grams per day. However, a woman expecting multiples needs an increased amount. While you should discuss your specific requirements with your doctor or nutritionist, many experts recommend that expectant mothers of multiples consume 100 to 150 grams of protein daily. Protein is not stored in the body, so it's important to replenish the supply by eating adequate amounts throughout the day, not just at dinner. Here are some protein-rich foods to stock up on:

- Eggs
- Cheese

- Yogurt
- Chicken breast
- Fish
- Lean meats such as turkey, ham, or roast beef
- Nuts such as almonds, walnuts, and cashews
- Peanut butter
- Tofu
- Soy milk products
- Beans

Keep Eating Those Carbs!

In addition to protein, your body needs an energy boost from complex carbohydrates. Pregnancy is not the time to jump on the low-carb-diet bandwagon! Carbohydrates help your body process the extra protein you're consuming and maintain your blood sugar. Just as with protein, it's important to choose the right source of carbohydrates.

There are two types of carbohydrates, simple and complex. Simple carbohydrates give a quick boost of energy from sugar, while complex carbohydrates release energy more slowly over time. Fruit is the preferred source of simple carbohydrates, rather than sugary treats such as candy, cake, or cookies, because of the added vitamins and nutrients it contains. Many fruits also have high water content, so they provide hydration as well as nourishment. Complex carbohydrates are found in many starchy foods, such as bread, cereal, pasta, potatoes, and rice, as well as some vegetables and legumes, such as beans and peas. Choose whole-grain starches for the added fiber they provide. A fiber-rich diet prevents constipation and can reduce your risk of contracting hemorrhoids.

Don't Forget Your Minerals and Vitamins

As you make food choices during your pregnancy, you should consider foods that provide vital minerals such as iron, calcium, and folic acid. While these substances are also available in the form of dietary supplements, you'll give your babies a better start if you ingest them naturally in the foods you eat. Calcium is essential in the creation of your babies' skeletal structure and also enhances heart, muscle, and nerve function. Although the most common source of calcium is dairy products, many green vegetables contain double or triple the amount. Arugula, spinach, and collard greens are excellent sources of calcium.

FACT

Calcium not only helps build your babies' bones and teeth, but it's also been proven to reduce the risk of pregnancy-induced hypertension and preeclampsia. It's good for Mom, too!

Many expectant moms of multiples experience anemia due to their increased blood volume during pregnancy. Because iron helps transport oxygen in the blood, it helps combat anemia. The problem with iron intake is that you not only have to take it in, but your body also has to absorb it properly. Some foods enhance iron absorption and others inhibit it, so food combinations are important. Dairy products, bran cereal, antacids, tea, and soda products can hinder absorption, but waiting about an hour after ingestion to eat iron-rich foods or take an iron supplement will reduce the inhibiting effects. Drinking orange juice may also help, since vitamin C helps convert iron into a form more easily absorbed by the body. Iron-rich foods include:

- Red meats
- Spinach
- Eggs
- Prunes
- Pumpkin seeds
- Soybeans

Folic acid is a B vitamin that is credited for dramatically reducing the risk of birth defects in the brain and spinal cord when taken prior to and during pregnancy. Folate, the natural form of the vitamin, is found in some food sources, such as black beans, asparagus, orange juice, spinach, peanuts, and romaine lettuce. Because of its benefits, some grain products, such as breads, cereals, and pastas, are now enriched with folic acid. However, to ensure that your intake is sufficient, pregnant mothers of multiples should also take a supplement or prenatal multivitamin that includes folic acid.

How Much Should I Eat?

In addition to selecting the right foods to eat during pregnancy, you have to think about how much you're eating. Remember, you are not just eating for two, as in a singleton pregnancy. You have to consume enough calories to sustain yourself as well as the two, three, or more developing fetuses.

Most pregnant women are advised to increase their daily caloric intake by about 13 percent. For most women, that's about 300 extra calories per day. That's not enough for mothers of multiples. Rather, they should aim for 300 extra calories *per baby* per day. That means mothers of twins need an additional 600 calories and mothers of triplets need to increase their intake by about 900 calories. With higher order multiples, it can be difficult to eat enough food to meet the demand; there are only so many hours in the day! Expectant mothers of quadruplets or more should discuss their specific dietary needs with their physician to determine the optimum caloric goal. Your caregiver can also help you come up with strategies to meet that goal.

ESSENTIAL

Studies have confirmed the benefits of early weight gain in pregnancy, so it's important to start increasing your food intake as soon as your multiple pregnancy is confirmed. A simple way to start is by consuming small mini-meals at snack time—mid-morning, afternoon, and evening. Then increase your caloric intake at meals by adding an additional serving of fruit, vegetable, or protein.

The Food Guide Pyramid

The USDA Food Pyramid gives recommendations for the type and amount of food that healthy individuals should consume each day, as shown in the following chart.

Fats, Oils, & Sweets
& White Starches
USE SPARINGLY

Meat, Poultry, Fish,
Dry Beans, Eggs, &
Nuts Group
1–5 SERVINGS

Milk, Yogurt, &
Cheese Group
1–2 SERVINGS

Vegetable Group
In Abundance

Fruit Group
2–3 SERVINGS

Whole Grain Food
& Plant Oils
AT MOST MEALS
6–11 SERVINGS

▲ The USDA Food Pyramid's dietary recommendations.

Expectant mothers of multiples are usually encouraged to aim for the higher number of servings in the range:

- Whole grains at every meal (bread, cereal, crackers, rice, or pasta)
- Abundant servings of colorful vegetables throughout the day
- 3 servings of a variety of fruits, not including fruit juices
- 3 servings of dairy products (milk, cheese, yogurt)
- 3–4 servings of protein from a variety of sources (meat, dry beans, eggs, seafood, nuts)

The USDA revised the Food Guide Pyramid in 2005; however, standards for expectant moms of twins, triplets, or more have not been clearly defined under the new guidelines. More information is available at *www.mypyramid.gov*. Always check with your physician for the most current dietary standards and how they apply to your particular health situation.

The Brewer Diet

The Brewer Diet for Pregnancy was developed by Dr. Thomas Brewer and originally published in the 1970s. It claims to prevent pregnancy complications such as intrauterine growth retardation (IUGR), preterm labor, and preeclampsia. In general, the Brewer Diet for Pregnancy advocates the following daily requirements:

- 4 servings of milk
- 2 eggs
- 6 servings of meat or vegetarian protein
- 2 servings of fresh, leafy green vegetables
- 5 servings of carbohydrates in the form of whole grain bread, starchy vegetables, or fruit
- 2 servings of vitamin-C-rich foods, such as citrus fruit or tomatoes
- 5 servings of fat or oil (butter, oil, mayonnaise)
- 1 serving of vitamin-A-rich food (orange-colored fruit or vegetables such as sweet potatoes or apricots)

Your doctor can help you decide whether this diet would be appropriate for your situation.

ALERT!

Follow your body's cues. In many cases, your body will seek to satisfy a nutritional need by signaling your brain with cravings. A craving for spinach or red meat may indicate a need for iron, while a strong desire for snacks like pretzels or potato chips may be a sign that your body needs more salt.

Nutritional Supplements

In order to obtain maximum nutritional benefits, your doctor may prescribe dietary supplements. Most experts agree that it is easiest for the body to utilize nutrients, vitamins, and minerals when they are obtained through foods, but during a multiple pregnancy, it may be necessary to ingest them in other forms. Your doctor or midwife will be able to advise you on the appropriate dosage and schedule; don't take any vitamins or supplements without consulting a medical professional.

Most women are advised to take a prenatal vitamin daily during their pregnancy, and many begin this regimen even before conception in order to give their baby an optimum start in life. Prenatal vitamin products are specifically designed to provide an extra boost of the vitamins and minerals that are most difficult to obtain through food, while minimizing the elements that can be dangerous to a developing fetus. Regular daily vitamin supplements may be too high in vitamin A, an excess of which has been linked to birth defects, or too low in important nutrients like folic acid and iron.

Folic acid, a B vitamin, is essential for the healthy development of a baby's spinal cord and brain. Taken prior to and early in pregnancy, it can help prevent up to 74 percent of neural tube defects, such as spina bifida and anencephaly.

Many expectant mothers of multiples experience iron deficiency, or anemia. Mothers of multiples are especially susceptible to this condition, so your doctor may routinely recommend an iron supplement in the second or third trimester. It is difficult to obtain sufficient amounts of iron, even with a healthy diet.

Unfortunately, supplemental iron can have some uncomfortable side effects. Constipation is a common complaint, but you can overcome the effects of it by increasing the amount of fiber in your diet. Drinking plenty of water helps, as well. Vitamin C enhances your body's ability to absorb iron, so wash down your daily dose with a glass of orange juice.

If you are underweight, or if you are losing weight due to loss of appetite or nausea, your doctor may advise you to augment your caloric intake with nutritional supplements. These products are available in a variety of flavors, usually in the form of a beverage or pudding snack. They are nutritionally balanced and calorie dense. If your doctor believes they are appropriate for your situation, he may recommend either a high-protein or high-calorie supplement, or perhaps a combination of both. They are not intended to replace food, but rather to increase your nutritional intake in order to maximize the healthy development of your babies.

Your doctor may also prescribe other supplements, such as calcium, magnesium, zinc, vitamin B, or vitamin D, depending on your individual needs. Of course, you should never take any dietary supplements without discussing them with your physician first. And always follow the recommended dosage amounts. Too much of a good thing is not good!

The Importance of Fluids

Eating right is a good start, but you also have to think about what you drink. Dehydration poses risks to the babies, including preterm labor, as well as causing constipation and other complications for mom. Getting your fill of liquids is every bit as important as fueling up on food.

During pregnancy, the blood volume in your body increases, nearly doubling its non-pregnant amount. Your body needs fluid to produce all that extra blood. Thus, good hydration improves your circulation, making you feel better and enhancing the development of your babies. You also require fluid to replenish the amniotic fluid surrounding the babies in your womb. If you're not drinking sufficiently, your body will leach the fluid from other systems. Ultimately, you can end up feeling lethargic, have dry, itchy skin, and become constipated.

Dehydration can also prompt the onset of preterm labor. In fact, rehydration is often one of the first lines of defense against early contractions. You can minimize the risk of preterm labor, and possibly keep yourself out of the hospital, by drinking plenty of fluids.

Most pregnant women are advised to drink six to eight glasses of liquid a day. However, that's if they're having one baby! Moms of multiples should strive for about sixty-four ounces, or about eight eight-ounce glasses. You may find it difficult to fill up on fluid. Try these tips and tricks:

- Drink a glass of water before each meal, then refill a glass to sip while you eat.
- Add slices of lemon or lime to flavor plain water.

- Try sparkling waters; the bubbles make them as refreshing as soda.
- Keep a full water bottle next to your bed so that you can sip in the night and first thing in the morning.
- Carry a bottle of water in the car and take a drink at every stoplight.
- Size up: Pour larger glasses or purchase larger bottles.

QUESTION?

Are any fluids okay, or do I have to drink water?
Water is the best choice. It provides all the elements your body needs without the high calories and added sugars of soda or juice. Sodas also contain phosphorus, too much of which can interfere with the body's ability to process calcium and iron. Caffeinated beverages can actually serve to dehydrate you as you drink them, and alcoholic beverages should be avoided entirely during your pregnancy.

If you aren't sure whether you're drinking enough, check your urine. The lighter the color of your urine, the more hydrated you are. If it's a dark yellow color, you could be dehydrated.

Exercise and Activity

Regular exercise is a vital part of a healthy lifestyle, but during a multiple pregnancy, it can sometimes cause extra stress and strain on your body. You should work with your health-care provider to determine an exercise plan that will incorporate the benefits while minimizing the risks.

Should You Exercise?

If you were active prior to your pregnancy, you may be able to continue your routine. However, pregnancy is not the time to start training for a marathon. Your body is simply too busy building babies to undertake strenuous activity. You should focus your exercise effort on activities that enhance your circulation, strengthen your muscle tone, and help you relax.

Make sure you're exercising for the right reasons during your pregnancy. Don't let weight management be the motivation behind your workout. Instead, focus on overall health for you and the babies.

Follow your doctor's advice. During the first trimester, you may be able to follow your normal, pre-pregnancy fitness routine, as long as you're aware of your need for extra supplemental calories and hydration. However, as the weeks pass, you will likely be advised to avoid exercise that compromises your pregnancy or puts you at risk for complications. Strenuous exercise can cause you to overheat or become dehydrated. You should avoid any high-impact activity that puts extra pressure on the pelvic floor and can induce preterm labor, such as running or aerobic dancing. Any exercises that strain the abdominal muscles, such as sit-ups or leg lifts, can be damaging during pregnancy. As your uterus grows, your body's center of gravity changes. You may find that your sense of balance is affected, making you unsteady and at higher risk for spills and tumbles.

If you are expecting higher order multiples, exercise may simply be too risky. The combined weight of the babies increases very quickly, making it more difficult for you move easily. Meanwhile, additional exercise may compromise your attempts to sustain high levels of caloric intake, since exercise just burns up calories that would be better applied toward the babies.

Exercise Options

With your doctor's blessing, swimming can be an ideal exercise during your pregnancy. If you have access to a pool, take advantage of it! Swimming provides a cardiovascular workout and feels very refreshing. If swimming laps isn't appealing, consider other water-based exercise options. The buoyancy of the water allows you to move comfortably and reduces strain on your body, creating an optimal exercise environment for a pregnant woman.

Walking is another excellent exercise option. It's free, doesn't require any special equipment, and is easily accessible. You can set your own pace and adjust your level of intensity according to how you're feeling. You can walk outside in fair weather, or head inside to a shopping mall when it's too hot, too cold, or rainy.

FACT

With any exercise program, be sure to wear supportive clothing and proper footwear. Your feet will swell and enlarge during pregnancy; you may have to invest in a larger pair of sneakers!

Gentle stretching exercises are also beneficial. Pregnancy yoga classes are available in many locations. The mental relaxation fostered by yoga can be especially soothing. Of course, check with your doctor before participating in a yoga routine, and ensure that the class instructor is fully qualified. To find a good class in your area, inquire at the hospital where you plan to deliver or check with your local mothers of multiples organization.

Rest and Relaxation

Even if you realize that sleep will be a precious commodity after the babies are born, you may be surprised at how difficult it is to sleep through the night during pregnancy. Between the physical discomforts of heartburn and leg cramps, and anxiety about what's ahead, you may have trouble settling down at night. However, a good night's rest is one of the best gifts that you can give your body—and your babies.

Overcoming Sleep Disturbances

Throughout your pregnancy, there are a variety of issues that cause physical discomfort or otherwise interfere with sleep. To combat sleep disturbances, or outright insomnia, try to pinpoint the cause of your restlessness. Do you wake up because you need to urinate? Are you unable to find a comfortable sleeping position due to your growing girth? Are you plagued by leg cramps, snoring, or heartburn?

In the first and last trimester, your pregnancy may impose on your bladder. In the early weeks, pressure from your expanding uterus may send you running to the bathroom frequently throughout the day—and night. In the final days, no matter how far you grow out and around, things are pretty crowded inside you, and your bladder has nowhere else to go. Unfortunately, there's not much you can do to alleviate the condition when it wakes you up at night, except to reduce the amount of fluid that you drink as it gets closer to bedtime. You'll still need to drink plenty during the day, however.

ALERT!

Sleeping pills are not recommended for pregnant women. They can cause birth defects, such as cleft palate. Talk to your doctor before taking any sleep aids, even herbal remedies.

Leg cramps and backaches are also uncomfortable side effects of pregnancy. Your muscles are working overtime because of the added weight of the babies. They can protest loudly—and painfully—by seizing up or spasming in the night. A lack of calcium or phosphorous in your diet can make the problem worse. A handheld massage unit may help alleviate the tension in your legs, but if the problem persists, you may wish to consult your doctor. She may be able to recommend a pain relief product that is safe to take during pregnancy.

Heartburn

It's not just your drinking habits that can keep you up at night; what you eat has an effect as well. Heartburn is a common complaint among the sleepless. As your uterus expands to accommodate two or more babies, digestive acids from your stomach are forced northward, causing a burning sensation in your digestive tract. It won't hurt the babies, but it can make you uncomfortable, especially when you're lying down.

To combat heartburn at night, avoid common triggers like spicy, fried, or fatty foods. Don't eat large quantities of food close to bedtime. Drink plenty of water with and between meals. Altering your bed's incline can also help. Raise the head of your bed by about six inches to allow gravity to keep your stomach in check. If all else fails, talk to your doctor about over-the-counter heartburn remedies. Many moms find that keeping a bottle of chewable tablets on the nightstand provides quick access to relief when heartburn strikes in the middle of the night.

Tossing and Turning

Even if you're exhausted, it can be nearly impossible to get comfortable enough to fall asleep when you're pregnant, especially if you are accustomed to sleeping on your stomach or back. You may feel like a beached whale in bed, floundering to find a comfortable position. Your expanding body needs support, and extra pillows can provide it. There are specially designed pregnancy pillows on the market, but if you want to spare the expense, experiment with extra bed pillows or throw cushions. Many women find that sleeping with a pillow between their knees or at the small of their back provides comfort. Others use pillows to prop their belly.

FACT

The recommended sleeping position in pregnancy is lying on the left side. It prevents your body weight from settling on your liver and optimizes the circulation of blood from your heart to your lower body.

If you simply can't get comfortable in bed, head for the living room. Many mothers find rest in a large reclining chair. It's easier to get in and out of when they need to get up to use the bathroom, and you don't have to worry about disturbing your partner. And it can simply be easier to relax in a reclined position than lying flat in bed.

The Need to Nap

Pregnancy can wreak havoc on your sleep habits. There may be occasions, especially in the first trimester, when the sedative effect of progesterone makes you incredibly sleepy during portions of the day when you need to be wide awake. Likewise, you'll sometimes find yourself wakeful and alert in the middle of the night if the babies or your bladder are particularly active.

Take advantage of opportunities to nap when you can. Short periods of rest do provide some restorative benefits. You may find it refreshing to catch a catnap the day after a restless night. Listen to your body's cues. Give it rest when you feel tired.

Things to Avoid

While there are certain things that you can do enhance your health during pregnancy, there are many things that you should *not* do in order to assure the safety of your developing babies. Certainly, there are some activities, such as excessive drinking and smoking, that are inadvisable at any time, but the potential harm to two, three, or more developing individuals makes these actions inexcusable during pregnancy. However, other seemingly harmless things that were part of your life before you were pregnant may pose a danger now that you are expecting twins or more.

For example, soaking in a hot tub should be avoided during pregnancy. Studies have shown a connection between hot tub use and miscarriage in the first trimester. In addition, soaking in a 100-plus-degree hot tub can cause a body's internal thermostat to rise and overheat, a dangerous condition for the fetuses.

That morning jolt of caffeine from coffee may be a cherished routine when you're not pregnant, but you may want to consider cutting back or going without while you are. Although moderate amounts of caffeine aren't necessarily harmful, studies have shown an association with stillbirth, birth defects, and other complications. Caffeine, found in coffee and some teas and sodas, stimulates your heart rate and metabolism. That can put stress on your body, and your babies. Your doctor can advise you as to how much is too much.

Caffeine can hamper your ability to absorb iron by as much as 40 percent if you drink a caffeinated beverage within one hour of a meal. That's a factor worth considering when you're already at risk for iron deficiency.

Medications and Herbs

The shelves of pharmacies overflow with over-the-counter medications and remedies for every known condition. Usually you wouldn't think twice about taking aspirin for a headache or a decongestant for a cold. However, you would never give these drugs to an infant, which is basically what you're doing when you take medications during your pregnancy. Any over-the-counter drugs should be approved by your doctor. If you are taking prescription drugs, your health-care provider will review your situation and make a recommendation as to whether it is safe to continue their use during pregnancy.

The popularity of herbal remedies to treat common ailments has risen in recent years. Be wary about their use during your pregnancy; you're not only administering them to yourself, but they will also impact your babies' well-being. Don't be misled into thinking that "natural" or nonmedical approaches are necessarily neutral; they may have harmful consequences. Always consult a medical provider before taking any kind of herbal product, including herbal teas, when you're pregnant.

Unsafe Foods

Listeriosis is an infection caused by eating foods that contain the *listeria* bacteria. It's not a terribly dangerous condition for most adults, but can have devastating effects on fetuses or newborns. You can reduce your risk of contracting such an infection by avoiding certain foods. Soft cheeses, including Brie, Camembert, feta, Roquefort, and asadero, should only be eaten if they have been cooked by boiling or broiling until they are bubbly. You can also minimize your risk by properly handling other foods that are likely to be contaminated with listeria. These include any foods that have been precooked and then refrigerated, such as hot dogs or deli-style luncheon meats. Cooking these foods will kill the bacteria, so they are safe to eat after they have been thoroughly reheated.

FACT

About one-third of all cases of listeriosis occur in pregnant women. They are particularly susceptible because pregnancy hormones cause changes to their immune system. Women who are pregnant are about twenty times more likely to contract the disease.

Despite its reputation as a delicious source of nutrition, some seafood is also potentially dangerous during pregnancy with multiples. Toxic levels of methyl mercury can be found in some types of predator fish, including shark, swordfish, tile fish, and king mackerel. Mercury can damage the developing fetuses' nervous system. That doesn't mean that you can't enjoy seafood while you're pregnant. Check with your doctor about the types of fish to avoid, and enjoy other varieties in moderation.

Cat Litter

You don't have to give up your kitty while you're expecting, but stay away from the litter box. Toxoplasmosis is a parasite that can be contained in cat waste. If you have a cat, you may already have been exposed to it, and it's not harmful to most adults. But it can cause health problems for unborn babies, so you want to limit your exposure.

Handling your cat won't bring you in contact with the parasite, but you should avoid coming in contact with feline feces. Have someone else clean the litter box while you're pregnant to minimize the risk. It's not likely to be a chore that you relish doing anyway!

Secondhand Smoke

Even if you don't smoke, the dangerous effects of tobacco can still impact your babies. Secondhand smoke, also known as passive smoke, is the combination of exhalations from a smoker and smoke from their burning cigarettes, and it can be harmful to developing fetuses. Babies exposed to secondhand smoke are smaller and more likely to be born prematurely; with your multiples already at risk for these conditions, you don't want to heighten the odds. Passive smoke increases the risk of asthma and cancer, and children of smokers often exhibit increased irritability.

Stay away from smokers while you're pregnant. Keep your home smoke-free; if you have family members who smoke, ask them not to smoke inside while you're pregnant. (Better yet, ask them to stop altogether!) Avoid the smoking section of public places such as restaurants and shopping centers.

Chapter 8

Your Medical Care

During your pregnancy with twins, triplets, or more, your medical care is crucial to ensuring a healthy outcome for you and your babies. If you have led a relatively healthy life up until this point, you may find the medical interventions somewhat overwhelming. Throughout the course of your pregnancy, you will be poked and prodded and probed. Educating yourself about the medical aspects of multiple birth will help you cope, and prepare you for an optimal pregnancy and birth experience.

What's Different When There's More Than One?

When you discovered that you were having twins, triplets, or more, you probably realized instantly that your pregnancy would be in a different category. Pregnancy accords a special status—people give up their seats on buses for you!—but now you are more than "just pregnant." You have been elevated to an entirely different status.

But what is really different? When all is said and done, the ultimate difference between having a singleton and having multiples is extra babies. There may be problems and complications along the way, but for the majority of cases, the end result is healthy children. While you can't ignore the increased risks inherent in a multiple pregnancy, you have to recognize them for what they are—they are possibilities, not certainties.

FACT

According to one study, the medical costs of a twin pregnancy were found to be five times higher than those of a singleton pregnancy. The costs escalate with each additional baby.

However, because of the risks, you are likely to receive more attention and intervention from your medical caregivers. You will be scheduled for more frequent checkups and assessments with your doctor or midwife. That is not necessarily a bad thing. The extra monitoring means that you are more likely to catch potential problems and may have access to more effective treatments.

While you may experience heightened symptoms, not every woman has extreme morning sickness or an extra dose of back pain. The amount of agony does not increase exponentially with each baby. Think about it this way: Although you might have to put up with some additional inconvenience and discomfort, you are condensing the trauma into one pregnancy, rather than spreading it out over several years!

Finding the Right Doctor

Choosing a medical practitioner is one of the most important decisions that you will make during your pregnancy, affecting many aspects of your experience. You will spend many hours in this person's office in the next few months, and your choice will ultimately impact how, where, and when your babies make their entry into this world. You should examine all your options and put some thoughtful consideration into your decision.

Depending on how your pregnancy was initiated, you may already be under the care of a doctor, nurse, or midwife. If your multiples were conceived as a result of fertility enhancements, your reproductive specialist may have referred you to a caregiver. Or maybe you have already been seeing a family practitioner, doctor, or midwife during your pregnancy, but now that you know you are having more than one baby, aren't sure if you need more specialized care.

ALERT!

Finding out that you're expecting twins or multiples may mean a change of course for your medical care. The right doctor for your singleton pregnancy may not be the best option for your multiples. Be flexible about the change to give your babies the best possible care.

Family Practitioner

Before you were pregnant, you probably had a family doctor that you visited when you were sick or hurt. It is wonderful to have a medical professional with whom you are comfortable and familiar, and who knows your history and background. Many doctors in family practice also provide prenatal care for pregnant women and some even deliver babies.

While that is fine for routine pregnancies, having twins or more puts you in a different class of risk, and your family doctor may not be able to provide the best care for you and your babies. You will have to weigh your options; are you more comfortable in the care of a trusted physician with whom you have a prior relationship or are you better off with a specialist who is experienced in multiple birth? If you choose to remain in the care of your family practitioner, be sure that he has had plenty of prior experience with multiple pregnancy. This is only a safe option if you are having twins (not more) and your pregnancy remains fairly free of problems, as family doctors don't usually have access to the kinds of specialized equipment required to treat complications.

Ob-Gyn

The most common choice for pregnancy and birth care is an obstetrician-gynecologist, or ob-gyn. This type of doctor specializes in care of women. Obstetrics focuses specifically on birth and the associated issues of pregnancy, labor, delivery, and postpartum care, while gynecology is the branch of medicine dealing with diseases and routine care of the female reproductive system. The certification of ob-gyn covers both areas, but some doctors prefer to specialize only in gynecology and choose not to deliver babies.

You may have been seen for an annual checkup or routine care by a gynecologist prior to your pregnancy, but in the event that she does not participate in childbirth, you will have to find an alternative.

After medical school and four years of residency training in women's health, ob-gyn physicians must pass written and oral tests to become certified by the American Board of Obstetrics and Gynecology. Some doctors pursue additional certification to become a Fellow of the American College of Obstetricians and Gynecologists; they are identified by the acronym FACOG after their title. Within the field, some ob-gyn practitioners specialize in maternal-fetal medicine; these individuals are most experienced with high-risk pregnancies and best equipped to handle the associated complications.

Perinatologist

A perinatologist is even more specialized than an ob-gyn, with extra qualifications specifically in handling high-risk pregnancies. Perinatologists undergo training beyond the regular obstetrics residency, spending three additional clinical years in research and patient care. They are the top professionals for diagnosing and treating medical conditions that threaten the health of the mother or babies during pregnancy. Because they deal with high-risk situations, perinatologists often have a richer depth of experience with multiple birth. In addition, they are usually associated with leading hospital facilities and have access to the latest and greatest technology for diagnosing and treating the conditions that might affect your babies' health.

Exploring Options:
Midwives, Doulas, and Home Births

For centuries, it was midwives, rather than doctors, that assisted women with the process of giving birth. Before the advent of medical technology, midwives delivered plenty of sets of twins and, although the rate of infant mortality was quite high, occasional sets of higher order multiples as well. Recent trends in childbirth steer back toward a more natural, less medical experience.

Midwives

Many women are returning to the use of midwives for care during pregnancy and childbirth. A certified nurse-midwife (CNM) is licensed to practice after obtaining a degree in nursing and completing specialized training as a midwife. These women generally provide a more individualized approach to care, focusing on the patient's goals for her childbirth experience.

Midwives are not usually equipped to handle high-risk pregnancies and deliveries. Because of the risks associated with multiples, expectant mothers are often discouraged from considering a midwife. However, the advantages of utilizing the services of a midwife are underestimated. Many CNMs are fully capable of handling the needs of uncomplicated twin deliveries, and occasionally even higher order multiples.

FACT

In 2002, midwife-attended births accounted for 10 percent of all vaginal deliveries in the United States. Many midwives claim lower rates of infant mortality and fewer cesarean births than doctors. (Keep in mind that midwives will refer most complicated or high-risk cases to specialists.) They are often much less expensive, as well.

Any midwife who truly values her patient's well-being will work in conjunction with an obstetrician or perinatologist who can offer specialized care in the event that it is warranted. If you are considering a midwife's services during your pregnancy with multiples, ensure that she can readily provide access to other health-care professionals if you encounter any complications.

Doulas

If your heart is set on a midwife but your body just won't cooperate, a doula may be a good compromise. A doula is a professional birth assistant who acts as your advocate in a medical setting. She is trained in the physiology of birth and is also equipped to help you cope with the emotional aspects of childbirth. She will provide support, physical comforting, and an objective perspective about the events surrounding the birth of your multiples. Studies have shown that women who use the services of a doula have faster labors, decreased use of epidurals, and fewer c-sections.

You can hire a doula to attend you during labor, delivery, and even after the babies are born. Many doulas are trained as lactation consultants and can assist with breastfeeding. They can also provide an extra set of hands when caring for your new infants. They may even be available prior to delivery, offering their services as a caregiver if you are on bed rest.

You will want to interview and hire a doula long before you are ready to deliver. Discuss her credentials, training, and background, and be sure to ask about her birth philosophies. Inquire about her specific experience with twins or multiples. Doulas certified by the International Childbirth Educators Association (ICEA) have completed a professional training program. Many hospitals will only let certified doulas attend a birth, especially if a cesarean section is required, so this certification should be an important factor in making your choice.

ALERT!

Doulas aren't cheap. They can charge from a few hundred to over a thousand dollars, depending on how long you utilize their services. Despite the benefits, few insurance companies will cover the cost. The extra support may be well worth the expense, however, especially for parents of multiples.

Home Birth

Although rare in the modern era of medicalized childbirth, recent years have seen a trend toward the return of home births. Some women prefer the familiar setting of their family home as the location for childbirth. While it is not particularly advisable, and probably outright dangerous in the case of higher order multiples, some women may want to pursue this option for delivery of their twins. If this is your desire, your best approach is to locate a midwife who is supportive of your plans, and who will work in conjunction with a doctor to provide backup care in the event of an emergency.

Making the Choice

With many options to choose from, how will you know what is best for you during your pregnancy? Ultimately, that decision will be based on your comfort level and the conditions of your pregnancy. If you are in good overall health, are having twins, and are committed to eating right and taking good care of yourself, you may be most comfortable with a doctor or midwife. However, if you are having higher order multiples, you should probably receive care from a specialist.

In some cases, you can have the best of both worlds. In many cities, group practices offer access to a variety of medical professionals within the same setting. You can visit a midwife or nurse practitioner for routine check-ups, see a perinatologist for ultrasound screening, and have an obstetrician deliver the babies.

FACT

Banner Good Samaritan in Phoenix, Arizona, has become one of the leading hospitals for high-risk multiple pregnancies. Women from all over the country travel to Arizona to receive care. In 2003 alone, the facility welcomed thirty-three sets of triplets, five sets of quadruplets, and two sets of quintuplets.

As multiple births become more common, some facilities are establishing "twin clinics" to address the specific needs of moms of multiples. These programs are more readily available in large cities and teaching hospitals, but are becoming more prevalent all over the country. They provide the advantage of centralized access to care focused exclusively on the unique aspects of a multiple pregnancy and delivery. However, the cost of their services is not always covered by insurance, and some women feel that the level of medical intervention is unnecessarily excessive for uncomplicated pregnancies.

In choosing a doctor, you should consider several things. Many times, your options may be narrowed or limited by your insurance coverage. No one wants to put a price on their babies' well-being, but the fact remains that medical care for pregnancy and birth is extremely expensive, even more so with multiple babies. If your insurance will pay for care from one doctor, but not from another, and both are equally qualified, then by all means choose a doctor associated with your insurance plan.

When making your choice, consider the physician's practice in addition to the individual. Is the office conveniently located? You will spend quite a bit of time there; toward the end of your pregnancy you will likely visit at least once a week. Does it have facilities for sonography and lab testing or do you have to go elsewhere? What hospital is your doctor affiliated with? Is it the best choice in the event that you or the babies have to receive long-term care? Who will handle your case if your choice of doctor or midwife is unavailable? These are all important questions. Make sure the answers to them satisfy your needs when considering your options.

Finally, consider your personal intuition as you make your choice. While you want the best possible care for your pregnancy, you also want a medical setting where you feel enabled to ask questions, receive adequate answers to those questions, and participate in your care as a partner.

Your Prenatal Care

During your pregnancy with multiples, and even after your babies are born, you will spend plenty of time in your health-care provider's office. Knowing what to expect during these visits will help you make the most of your time and ensure that you receive the best possible care for you and your babies.

The Initial Visit

Your first visit is a time to establish a relationship with your doctor and set the tone for the next nine months. You should call to schedule a visit as soon as you suspect that you are pregnant. If you've been receiving treatment from a reproductive specialist, they may continue to monitor you for a period of time after conception and advise you as to when you should arrange for prenatal care.

During the first visit, the doctor, nurse, or midwife will spend some time obtaining your medical history. Be prepared to delve deep into your medical background and to answer plenty of questions about your past illnesses, your family history of disease, and your lifestyle. The father-to-be won't escape the interrogation, either. It is important to establish his history as well, as it could impact the babies.

Before your visit, spend some time investigating your medical background. Ask relatives about their health history, so that you are fully prepared to answer any questions. Be especially aware of any genetic or inherited disorders, such as hemophilia or mental retardation, and any incidences of pregnancy loss or infant death.

You will be given a comprehensive physical exam, assessing your overall health. You will be weighed and measured, and your blood pressure will be monitored. You may receive a breast exam, and will most likely be given a pelvic exam, complete with a Pap smear. You may be asked to give a urine sample for analysis. You will have blood drawn, or will be scheduled for a visit to a lab at another site. Analysis of your blood will assess many different elements:

- Presence of HCG (human chorionic gonadotropin), a pregnancy hormone
- Blood type
- Hemoglobin and hematocrit (red blood cell count)
- Rh factor (rhesus)
- Antibody screening
- Rubella titer (German measles)
- Hepatitis B

Some doctors will screen for other conditions as well, such as immunity to varicella (chickenpox), HIV, toxoplasmosis, sickle-cell anemia, cystic fibrosis, and Tay-Sachs and other genetic disorders.

Your initial visit can be an exciting experience. In some cases it is a confirmation that you are indeed pregnant, or a revelation that you are expecting more than one. Your due date will be ascertained so that you can start anticipating the arrival of your new family members.

Future Visits

Every doctor or midwife has her own prescribed schedule of care for pregnant mothers of twins or more. Generally, you can expect to see the doctor more often when you are carrying more babies, and the frequency of your visits will increase as you go further along in your pregnancy. A typical schedule would look something like this:

- Initial visit between six and eight weeks; an ultrasound may be performed
- Monthly visits at twelve, sixteen, and twenty weeks

- Comprehensive ultrasound assessment at twenty weeks
- Visits twice a month after twenty weeks
- Weekly visits after twenty-eight weeks with nonstress testing, biophysical profiling, and other assessments

Depending on your progress, more frequent visits may become necessary until you deliver.

Don't underestimate the importance of personality; while you may not like every doctor or nurse you deal with, you should have confidence and trust in their ability to treat you and your children.

Choosing a Pediatrician

In addition to maternal medical care, you'll need to choose a caregiver for your multiples after they're born. If you have older children, you may already have a pediatrician or family practitioner. That individual can probably serve your needs for your new arrivals as well. However, you may want to consider some of the unique needs of multiples. It is helpful to have a doctor for your infants who has previous experience with twins or multiples, although it's not as crucial as during pregnancy.

Once your babies have arrived, they should be treated as individuals, and you'll want doctors who are qualified to handle their individual issues. If your babies are born prematurely or have special needs after birth, they will be treated in the hospital by a neonatologist, a specialist who treats infants with serious illnesses, injuries, or birth defects. However, most newborns only require a pediatrician, a doctor who specializes in treating babies and children. Ask your fellow parents of twins or multiples for recommendations. They'll give a glowing endorsement of doctors who are good candidates, and you'll know to steer clear of any who generate complaints.

There are some further criteria to consider when choosing a doctor for your multiples. These are mostly issues of convenience, not qualifications, but they may weigh in your decision.

Convenience

Choose a doctor who practices in a location and setting that is easily accessible. You'll be paying plenty of visits to his office in the next few years; minimize the hassles as much as you can. When you visit the office, check out the facilities. Is it easy to park and enter the building? Can you easily negotiate the entry, doorways, and stairways or elevator with a stroller or with your hands full? Are the office staff friendly and helpful?

In addition, find out the practice's policies. What happens after hours? Do they offer telephone support, such as an Ask-A-Nurse service? What if your doctor is unavailable? Are there partners or nurses whom you can see as an alternative?

FACT

Some pediatricians will offer a discount on well-baby care for multiples, perhaps a percentage off the charge for the second, third, or fourth baby. It doesn't hurt to ask!

Philosophy

When you interview potential doctors, find out their stance on parenting issues that are important to you, such as breastfeeding, family bed, immunizations, and circumcision. Only a face-to-face interview will reveal whether you are compatible with a doctor. It's important that you feel comfortable with her personality, and that you trust her ability to care for your children. You should not feel intimidated or rushed when you ask questions. Finally, you should get a sense that the doctor respects your intuition as a parent.

Chapter 9

E **Setting Up the Nursery**

One of the most exciting and fun ways that parents prepare for a new addition to the family is by creating the baby's room. For parents of multiples, who are expecting two or more, the process can present some extra challenges, but is every bit as rewarding. There is no specific formula to follow; depending on your home's space allocation, you may choose to put each child in his or her own room, designate a single room for all of them, or even create a "nursery niche" in a section of an existing room.

Cribs: One, Two, or More?

One of the biggest decisions parents of multiples will make about their babies concerns sleeping arrangements. Cribs are a big-ticket item in the nursery; not only do they consume a lot of floor space in a room, but they can also consume a big chunk of the budget!

Initially, you won't necessarily need an individual crib for every baby. Two or even three infants can easily share a sleeping space during the first few months. Instead of a crib, you may prefer to keep the babies close at hand by having them sleep with you, or nearby in a bassinet, cradle, portable crib, or Moses basket. Eventually, however, you'll want to provide a designated, segregated spot for each baby in order to ensure secure and uninterrupted sleep for everybody. Once the babies are old enough to roll or scoot around, they can disturb each other, and that's the time to invest in additional cribs.

FACT

There are some bed options designed specifically for twins, but their cost and space demands may make them prohibitive for most families. Baby Trilogy, Inc. sells wedge-shaped cribs that, when placed together, form a semi-circular unit for twins. They retail for close to $1,000 and require special bedding products at an additional cost.

Crib Safety Considerations

When choosing cribs for your babies, follow established safety guidelines, such as those developed by the U.S. Consumer Product Safety Commission. They recommend

- A firm, tight-fitting mattress so babies can't get trapped between the mattress and the crib
- No missing, loose, broken, or improperly installed screws, brackets, or other hardware on the crib or mattress support
- No more than $2^3/8$ inches (about the width of a soda can) between the crib slats so a baby's body can't fit through the slats; no missing or cracked slats

- No corner posts over $1/16$ inch high so a baby's clothing can't catch
- No cutouts in the headboard or footboard so a baby's head can't get trapped

For mesh-sided cribs and playpens, look for

- Mesh less than ¼ inch in size, smaller than the tiny buttons on a baby's clothing
- Mesh with no tears, holes, or loose threads that could entangle a baby
- Mesh securely attached to the top rail and floor plate
- Top rail cover with no tears or holes
- If staples are used, none that are missing, loose, or exposed

Choices, Choices

Another factor to consider when choosing cribs is longevity. Many families find it convenient to keep twins or more sleeping in cribs much longer than they would a singleton, perhaps even up to the age of three. In that case, the multiples may move right into—pardon the pun—twin beds. However, if you anticipate the need for an intermediate sleeping arrangement, toddler beds, with their protective railings and smaller mattresses, may be a viable option. Some crib models convert to toddler beds, extending their usefulness.

Staying in the Budget

Cribs and baby bedding can be expensive, with fancy solid wood items retailing for well over $1,000. When you're faced with buying two or more at the same time, it may make sense to investigate secondhand products. Local mothers of multiples clubs are a wonderful source for locating secondhand sets of cribs, as well as other baby equipment. When purchasing used products, be sure that they are in good condition and meet established safety guidelines.

Changing Table and Diaper Stations

A safe, sturdy changing station makes diaper duty more efficient. This is one piece of furniture that infant multiples will only use one at a time, but you may want to consider setting up multiple stations in convenient locations throughout the house. Be creative. A diaper station doesn't have to take the form of a traditional changing table; any sturdy furniture with a flat top, such as a dresser, can be transformed to accommodate your needs. Whatever you choose, make sure that it's a comfortable height and that your location provides sufficient but easily accessible storage. Stock your space with plenty of diapers, wipes, extra clothing, powders, creams, and lotions. Everything you need should be within arm's reach so that you never have to leave a baby unattended on the changing table. Finally, designate a convenient location for sanitary disposal of dirty diapers.

Bond with your babies while you're doing diaper duty. Use a gentle touch, make eye contact, and talk to each baby throughout the process. Hearing your voice enhances the babies' language development. If one baby fusses while his sibling is being attended to, calm him with soothing words, or even try singing!

When you set up your diaper station(s), be sure to provide a secure spot for the baby who's waiting his turn, since your hands and attention will be busy with the diaper process. In the babies' bedroom or nursery, it might be a crib. Other alternatives include a bouncy seat, bassinet, or playpen. Position it so that you can keep an eye on everyone, and won't ever have to turn your back on the baby who's being changed.

Other Useful Nursery Furniture

Complete your babies' nursery with additional furnishings that provide comfort for your family and storage for your children's things. Dressers with drawers and cabinets are handy for holding baby clothing and linens. Shelves with pretty baskets can contain tiny socks, sleepers, and diapers—you can never have enough storage space for extra diapers! Put away playthings in a toy bin or box.

Equip your nursery for daytime and nighttime usage. A comfortable chair, such as a glider or rocker, is a must. Parents of multiples will spend many tender moments in it; be sure you can reside there comfortably with all the babies at the same time! If you have the space, a small sofa or love-seat makes a convenient place for quick feedings or short snoozes while the babies sleep in their cribs.

Baby Monitors

Monitoring devices that allow you to listen to, or even watch, your babies without being in the room are an essential for parents of multiples. They provide you the freedom to roam around the house and a sense of security that your babies are safe and happy. It's almost like being in two places at the same time, something that parents of twins or more are often called on to be.

Baby monitors have two components: a base unit and a receiver. The base unit is the listening device, which is stationed near the babies. These units usually require a power source, so you'll probably have to position it near an electrical outlet. The signals detected by the base unit, such as sound or motion, are then transmitted to the receiver. A product with wireless receivers provides additional mobility, allowing you to move throughout the house without losing contact.

Some models have unique features such as motion sensors or remote controls. Some even operate like walkie-talkies, allowing you to communicate with your babies through the base unit. This can be a helpful feature for parents of multiples. Even if you're not able to enter the room because you are busy with another baby, the sound of your voice may be sufficient to calm an upset sibling.

Outfitting the Layette

Now that you have furniture for your babies' room, it's time to think about what you'll fill those dresser drawers with—what you'll soon use to cover their little bodies. A collection of clothing, blankets, bedding, and other "soft" items for babies is called a layette, although in recent years the term has been expanded to include all baby products. There are many layette checklists available, and you may be tempted to multiply the recommended amounts according to the number of babies you will have. That's not necessary, however, because multiples can share so many items.

FACT

As a general guideline, count on one and one-half times the suggested amounts of clothing and supplies for twins. Double the recommendations to meet the needs of triplets. Quadruplets will require two to three times the amount recommended for one baby. For quintuplets or more, count on three to four times the recommendations.

Baby Clothing

The baby clothing business is booming! Babies can be dressed to resemble their fashionable parents with designer togs in high style. But the practical fact of the matter is that baby clothes should be chosen for function and usefulness, and not just for their looks. Chances are those high-priced outfits will fall victim to spit-up stains, diaper disasters, or growth spurts before they've even cleared the credit card charge!

Clothing is a very popular gift for new families, and people especially like to buy cute ensembles for multiples. You'll likely be showered with outfits from well-meaning friends and relatives. Consider their generosity before you invest a great deal of your own money in clothing. When you do buy it, purchase with practicality in mind. Keep the tags attached until the babies are ready to wear each item, and save receipts so that you can easily return unneeded items.

You'll be surprised at how difficult it can be to anticipate clothing needs within size and season changes. In general, multiples tend to be a bit smaller than their singleton counterparts. They may wear newborn (0–3 months size) clothing for a longer period of time, especially if they are born early. However, some catch up very quickly and move into larger sizes within a matter of weeks.

To make it even more complicated, your multiples might not even wear the same sizes at the same time. There is often a weight and size discrepancy between twins, and not just among fraternal twins. Monochorionic identical twins that shared a placenta or had twin-to-twin transfusion syndrome can be vastly different sizes. Or a baby that experiences medical complications may not grow as fast as his healthy twin.

Dressing two or more infants can be a time-consuming chore, so choose clothing options that are easy to put on and take off. Snaps are preferable to buttons. Avoid shirts that have to be pulled on over the head; look for wide necks, snap fronts, or wrap styles. Likewise, don't struggle to pull on pants over wiggly baby legs. Snap crotches make diaper changes a breeze.

Used baby clothing is a bargain, and you'd be wise to seek out sources for it, such as consignment shops or multiples clubs sales. Check clothing for stains and tears before you buy, and be willing to reject overpriced items. If you shop smart you'll save a bundle. Better yet, chances are you can resell the items once your babies are through with them!

Getting Organized

Here's a checklist to help you itemize and organize your layette. Remember that these are only suggestions; your babies may require more or less.

For twins, expect to use:

- ❑ 8–10 T-shirts or Onesies for layering or wearing alone
- ❑ 6–8 lightweight sleepers (depending on the season)
- ❑ 6 blanket sleepers (depending on the season; fewer for warm-weather climates)
- ❑ 4 going-home outfits/special occasion outfits
- ❑ 4 hats
- ❑ 3 pairs of soft cotton mittens
- ❑ 6 pairs of socks/booties
- ❑ 4 sweaters/sacks/warm layers for winter
- ❑ 10 bibs (select a variety, including some waterproof items)

For triplets, plan on:

- ❏ 10 T-shirts or Onesies for layering or wearing alone
- ❏ 10–12 lightweight sleepers (depending on the season)
- ❏ 8 blanket sleepers (depending on the season; fewer for warm-weather climates)
- ❏ 6 going-home outfits/special occasion outfits
- ❏ 6 hats
- ❏ 5 pairs of soft cotton mittens
- ❏ 8 pairs of socks/booties
- ❏ 6 sweaters/sacks/warm layers for winter
- ❏ 15 bibs (select a variety, including some waterproof items)

Obviously, quadruplets or higher order multiples will require more clothing to meet their needs. Use the twins list as a base, and multiply the amounts to accommodate the number of babies.

FACT

All clothing and linens should be washed before the babies use them. Avoid fabric softener or other products that contain dyes or fragrances. Laundry products designed specifically for infants help prevent allergic reactions and skin conditions, and also help to preserve the protective quality of flame-retardant treatments.

Linens and Bedding

In addition to clothing and diapers, you'll need to stock your linen closet with several other items to accommodate your babies' needs for bedtime, bathtime, and beyond. Soft cotton receiving blankets are invaluable for keeping young infants swaddled, providing warmth, or creating a comfortable place to lie on the floor. They are also useful as cushioning when your babies are small and don't quite fit comfortably within the space of their stroller, bouncy seat, or infant car seat.

For the most part, crib bedding serves more of a fashion role than a functional one. Dust ruffles, pillows, and quilts are pretty, but not necessary. Bumper pads and mattress covers, on the other hand, protect your babies as well as your cribs! At a minimum, purchase at least one waterproof mattress protector per crib, plus one or two extras for quick changes. In addition, you'll want at least two sets of sheets per crib. If you're planning to use bassinets, cradles, or portable cribs, you'll need additional sheets for them as well.

Baby towels and washcloths are designed with babies' comfort in mind, but any kind of soft, absorbent cloth will work just fine when you bathe your babies. Hooded towels help keep babies' heads warm and dry after their bath.

You'll want an ample supply of burp or spit-up rags. Keep them handy during feedings and stash them throughout the house and in the diaper bag. Even if you're using disposable diapers, it pays to invest in a stockpile of cloth diapers for this purpose. They're soft, easy to clean, and inexpensive.

Double Decorating

After the furniture and layette items have been purchased, new parents can look forward to the excitement of decorating the nursery. There are many fun decorating schemes that will highlight your multiples' special status. Consider a Noah's Ark parade of two-by-two animals for twins, or The Three Bears for triplets. Cheerful colors will stimulate your babies, enhancing their visual development, while soothing pastel tones create a peaceful atmosphere. Just remember, by the time a baby is old enough to form an opinion about the décor, he is likely to have outgrown the blue bunnies that his parents chose before his birth. Don't be overly concerned about fashion, but rather focus your efforts on creating a functional room with an eye to the future. However you outfit it, your babies' nursery will be a special place where they feel the security of your love for them.

With practicality in mind, use washable paint products on the walls. Choose floor coverings that are easily cleaned and comfortable to crawl on. Lighting in a nursery is also very important. Look for controls that will allow you to dim or brighten the amount of light, even if your hands are full of babies or middle-of-the-night supplies.

Babyproofing

It will be several months after your babies are born before you actually have to lock every cabinet and hide all the breakables. However, it's never too early to start thinking about childproofing your home, and you certainly don't want to wait until it's too late, and pay the consequences of what could have been a preventable accident. Once you bring your babies home, free time will be harder to come by, and it may be too late to effectively evaluate your home's babyproofing needs.

If you have other children, you probably already have safeguards in place throughout your home. However, there are some extra precautionary measures to consider when you have twins or more. You've probably heard the old saying, "Two heads are better than one." Well, when it comes to outwitting parents' efforts to keep them out of trouble, that phrase is all too true about twins. Not only are there four hands for reaching and pulling, and four feet for climbing and running, but a twosome is always more creatively daring than one child on his own. And if two can wreak more havoc than one, just imagine what destruction three, four, or more can create!

ALERT!

The U.S. Consumer Product Safety Commission estimates that 2.5 million accidents occur annually in U.S. homes with young children. Most of those incidents could have been prevented with a few simple safety precautions.

You can't possibly anticipate every single danger or risk in your home. But you can try to minimize the potential for accidents or damage, both to your precious children and to your home's contents! Here are some general tips for preparing your home for multiples; you'll want to consult a more comprehensive source before your babies become mobile.

- **Store anything breakable or irreplaceable.** There's always time for knickknacks when your kids are grown. Why take a chance?
- **Keep all toxic chemicals, such as cleaning products or paints, out of reach.** Don't just move them to higher ground, but be sure the storage location has a lock or other obstacle. You don't want to discover your twins' innate talent for climbing to new heights when it's too late.
- **Keep your kids close to the ground.** Eliminate any situation that can create stair steps; secure dresser drawers, shelves, even dining room chairs.
- **Lock and double lock dangerous destinations.** You can buy "safety" locks or "childproof" hinges, but they often aren't enough to foil a team of twins. Double your efforts and use more than one safety precaution.
- **Soften edges.** Many accidents happen when kids come in contact with the sharp edges of furniture or walls, especially when babies are learning to crawl or walk. Bumpers or pillows can help soften the blow, or be on the safe side by removing furniture with sharp corners altogether.
- **Designate a safe zone.** Establish a place within your home that can be secured and freed of all possible hazards. It may be a playpen or crib for young babies, or a play yard or gated room for older ones. Then use it religiously. Never turn your back on your multiples unless they are in the zone.
- **Think like a kid.** Get down on the floor where your babies will play and check out the view, imagining every potential danger. Remove any small or detachable items that could be a choking hazard. Cover any electrical outlets and secure any electrical cords.

These changes to your home are temporary and worthwhile. At times, you may feel that you've been the victim of a home invasion, and that it has been overtaken by baby "stuff." Remember, this isn't a lifestyle you'll have to cope with forever.

Chapter 10

Buying Accessories and Equipment

The addition of twins or more to your family is going to have a big impact on your lifestyle, and your home must be ready to accommodate those changes. Any infant requires some specialized supplies and equipment, and you can bet that multiple babies need even more. But take heart. You don't necessarily have to double or triple all your supplies. There are some things that your babies can share, and some things that they won't need at all.

The Diaper Dilemma

The daunting task of diapering your babies is likely to be one of the most significant challenges you'll face as a parent of multiples. The good news is that it's only a temporary responsibility; eventually your kids will grow up and learn to use the bathroom. In the meantime, your goal is to devise an effective diaper system that makes the chore tolerable for everyone involved.

FACT

A family with twins is likely to perform nearly 5,000 diaper changes in the first year alone! Triplet parents should expect to serve close to 7,000 episodes of diaper duty and parents of quadruplets can look forward to 8,000 or more. In the first few months, each baby can go through as many as twelve diapers a day, so be sure to have at least a few dozen on hand before they're born.

Your first challenge is to confront the ultimate diaper dilemma: cloth or disposable? If you've already made this decision for previous children, there's no real reason to change your habits for multiples. Whatever satisfies your personal cost, conscience, and convenience qualifications is the right choice. For first-timers, here's an overview of the advantages and disadvantages of each option.

Disposable diapers offer the benefit of convenience. They are ready to use, easy to put on and take off, and require the diaperer to have minimal contact with the offensive contents. Used disposables go out with the trash and can be easily discarded when you're out and about. Absorbent materials mean that babies' bottoms may stay drier, cleaner, and more comfortable. The downside is that these diapers are costly (for both consumers and the environment). Even when bought in bulk at a discount, each diaper change can take about fifteen cents out of your pocket. When you tally the total over your babies' diaper lifetime, the cost easily reaches into the thousands of dollars.

Cloth diapers have their associated costs as well: namely, the water consumed to wash them. Unless you're willing to use organic cotton products and wash all the diapers yourself, your efforts have a negligible impact on the problem. The products and treatments used by professional diaper services arguably have just as many negative environmental consequences as disposable diapers. Likewise, a family's cost to use a diaper delivery and cleaning service rivals the price of disposables.

Cloth diapers do have several qualities to recommend them. New styles function much like disposables; the days of pinning bunches of cloth are long gone, and comfortable covers are available in a wide range of colors and fashions. The natural fabric of cloth may be more comfortable for babies with skin allergies or sensitivities, and may reduce occurrences of diaper rash in all babies.

Traditional diaper pails or Diaper Genies may be too small to accommodate your multiples' diaper output. If you like the convenience of these odor-reducing products, you may need to invest in two or three. They're useless without the odor-reducing liners, so be sure to stock up on these products too.

You'll need diapers on the go as well as at home. A well-stocked diaper bag will be your lifeline for managing your multiples out in the world. Keep it stocked with eight to ten diapers, a travel case of wipes, antibacterial hand cleaner, one change of clothes per baby, a blanket or pad, burp rags, and sealable plastic bags for disposing of dirty diapers.

Bottles and Feeding Accessories

Regardless of how you'll feed your babies, there are some basic supplies that you'll need. Even if you're not breastfeeding, you may find it useful to invest in a U-shaped nursing pillow or "Boppy." And even if you decide to nurse, it won't hurt to keep some bottles handy; they can be used to store pumped breast milk.

Bottle Basics

Bottles are available in a wide variety of shapes and sizes. Most bottles have three components: a vial for containing the fluid, a nipple that the baby sucks on to access the liquid, and a cap or ring that secures the nipple to the bottle. Infants, who only consume a few ounces of breast milk or formula during a feeding, require smaller containers than older babies or toddlers, who may drink eight or more ounces at a time.

The babies' age may also be a factor in choosing a nipple style. Newborns who are just learning to suckle may need a product with a slower flow to prevent the contents of the bottle from gushing out all over them. As they get older, hungry babies with a more powerful sucking reflex will prefer a nipple style that delivers the liquid more quickly. If you're using bottles to supplement breastfeeding, look for nipple styles that more closely resemble the human breast.

FACT

Some mothers prefer glass bottles for expressed breast milk due to concern over chemicals in plastic products. However, the risk of breakage with glass makes other parents steer clear.

Ultimately, the best choice is determined by personal preference—both yours and the babies'. Just as some adults would rather drink out of a crystal goblet than a plastic tumbler, babies sometimes prefer the feel and flow of a particular model of bottle. Even individual babies within a set of multiples will express a clear preference for one product over another. You may want to start off with a few varieties for your newborns, then stock up on supplies after you've established what works best.

Breast Pumps

Many mothers of multiples agree that a high-quality electric breast pump plays a valuable role when successfully breastfeeding multiples. Pumping immediately following a feeding or between feedings helps to establish a sufficient supply of breast milk for all the babies, and allows you to store the surplus for future feedings. Although inexpensive manual pumps exist, most women find that they simply aren't worth the hassle when they're pumping enough breast milk for more than one baby. Look for a model with a double pump, such as the Medela Pump In Style. It will allow you to extract milk simultaneously from both breasts, a precious timesaver for moms of multiples. They are not inexpensive, but worth the investment if you can afford it.

Some hospitals rent professional-grade equipment, but you'll need to evaluate whether the rental costs over time outpace the purchase price. The market for secondhand breast pumps is extensive; investigate the availability of a gently used model through your local parents of multiples organization or online.

ALERT!

Most other feeding accessories aren't needed right away. Your babies won't be able to sit up in high chairs until they're several months old; you can put off this purchase if you don't have the space in your kitchen or in your budget.

Choosing the Right Stroller

The stroller is perhaps the most crucial piece of equipment you will buy as a parent of multiples. Unless you plan to remain confined to your home until your children can walk themselves to school, you will need a good stroller to maneuver them through the world. Many families find that their stroller remains a convenient and safe method of transportation for several years, so it is worth investing in a quality product that will withstand some wear and tear. Think of it as a vehicle for your babies and give your purchase as much consideration as you would if you were buying a family car.

The Stroller Style Debate

Ask any parent of twins about their stroller, and they'll likely give you a passionate response as to why their model is the best choice available. However, there is no one perfect stroller; if there was, everyone would own it! Your perfect stroller is the one that meets your family's needs. It may be that there isn't a single stroller that fits your requirements, and you'll want to consider purchasing more than one for different types of outings.

There are two basic styles of strollers. Tandem, or stadium seating, strollers have seats arranged in a straight line, with one behind the other. The seats may both face forward or face each other. Side-by-side strollers, as their name implies, feature two adjacent seats. Each style has advantages and disadvantages, and according to informal polls, parents are pretty evenly split in their preferences.

Tandem Strollers

Tandem double strollers are more readily available because they aren't exclusively used for twins. Most models are actually designed for two singleton siblings. One seat may be a bit roomier or positioned higher to accommodate a toddler or preschool-aged child, while the other space is made for a smaller infant. Because they appeal to a broader market, they are more likely to come with handy accessories such as sunshades, drink holders, and snack trays.

◀ Tandem-style double stroller

Tandems are generally longer and more slender than side-by-side models. For this reason, some people find them easier to maneuver through narrow spaces, such as shopping center aisles and doorways. But there are also aspects of tandem strollers that don't work well with twins. In many models one of the seats, designed for an older child, does not fully recline. Until your babies' neck muscles develop sufficiently to hold their heads up, they need support. An upright seat is useless with younger infants and napping babies.

Many parents of twins rave about the new travel system of strollers that function in combination with infant carrier/car seats. Simply snap the seats into the stroller base and wheel your babies away. This convenient system eliminates the hassle of buckling and unbuckling—and buckling and unbuckling again—as you transfer your babies from the house to the car to the stroller and back.

Side-by-Side Strollers

Side-by-side strollers are a more traditional type of twin stroller. They operate most efficiently with two children of equal weight, and provide adequate leg- and headroom for both as they grow. One distinct advantage of the side-by-side style is that it positions both children with an equal viewpoint, which is the arrangement most twins seem to prefer.

Side-by-sides are wider than tandems, but have a shallower profile. That gives the stroller pusher more control and puts the babies in a closer arm's reach. Unfortunately many parents find their width hard to deal with in crowded or constricted locations, or when they need to go through single doorways or down narrow passageways.

◀ Side-by-side
double
stroller

Manufacturers have been slow to equip side-by-side models with some of the fancy features consumers expect. Storage baskets, bumpers, and sunshades are becoming more standard, but as of yet, there is not a side-by-side product that accommodates the handy travel system feature that works in conjunction with car seat/infant carriers.

One other potential problem to consider with side-by-side models: They put your twins in full view for the whole world to see. There is no chance of being anonymous! Twins, especially baby twins, attract a lot of attention when you take them out in public. It feels like everyone (especially perfect strangers) wants to look at them, compare their characteristics, interrogate their parents, and relate their own family's history of twinning.

FACT

If you think that being the center of attention will bother you, minimize it by sticking with a tandem-style stroller. They are more efficient at keeping the babies out of the public eye.

Choosing the Right Stroller for You

With advantages and disadvantages to both kinds of strollers, how can you possibly decide what you need? Should you just get two? Sounds like you've already adopted a multiple mindset! While that's often an effective solution to problems faced by parents of twins, it's not necessarily the answer when it comes to strollers. Consider the following when making your decision:

- **When will you use it?** Some strollers can accommodate infants, some are hardier for use with toddlers. Many families with twins find that they rely on a stroller long after their singleton counterparts; for longevity, select a model that is designed for children up to forty pounds.
- **Where will you use it?** All-terrain strollers are wonderful for jogging, hiking, or other outdoor activities, but they aren't very effective at maneuvering through tight indoor spaces such as office buildings or stores.
- **How will you use it?** Consider how your stroller will play a role in your everyday activities. Will you store it in your home? In the car? Will you use it to transport your babies to day care on a daily basis, or only for occasional jaunts to the park? Do you reside in a city location with crowded sidewalks and subways, or a rural environment with open, unpaved surfaces? Your specific circumstances will determine what kind of product will best serve your family.

Strollers for Triplets or More

If you're expecting triplets or more, your stroller options are more limited, and more costly. You'll have to carefully evaluate how you'll utilize the equipment, and anticipate whether the investment is worthwhile. You may wish to consider a combination of single and double strollers or a combination of strollers and other types of carriers, such as a sling or backpack.

Some stroller manufacturers do offer a triplet model, such as the Baby Jogger Triple Totter. This side-by-side model is best for open, outdoor spaces, with three seats that can also accommodate three children of different sizes. The Peg Perego Triplette offers stadium seating in a durable frame and fully reclining seats. Each of these products will set you back about $500 if purchased new.

Double Decker Stroller, Inc., a company started by a mom of multiples, makes an innovative stroller frame that accommodates infant carriers. The stroller is available in double and triple models. However, such products have a limited lifetime; when your babies outgrow the infant carriers (at 20 pounds or about one year of age), you'll need another stroller.

Custom-made strollers from Runabout are popular with parents of higher order multiples for their durability and value-added features. They can accommodate up to five children, including infants over ten pounds, with fully adjustable seats and a lightweight frame. They are individually made in the United States, are difficult to locate, and can retail for more than $1,000 for a quintuplet version, but they have excellent resale value and are very much in demand within the multiples community.

Seats, Carriers, and Swings

The market for baby products is jam-packed with gadgets and gizmos designed to contain, sustain, and entertain your babies. But since you'll end up providing at least two of each of these items, you'll need to focus on the ones that have been proven most useful.

Bouncy Seats

Bouncy seats, basically a sling covering a lightweight metal or plastic frame, are an inexpensive and convenient option for managing your multiple infants. They securely hold your babies when you need your hands free. Babies can eat in them, sleep in them, play in them, or wait their turn while their twin is being attended to. If you have a multi-level home, you'll want a set on every story.

ALERT!

Double and triple bouncy seats may seem like an essential for families with twins or triplets, but in reality, you'll do just as well with a combination of single seats. The single seats are lightweight enough to pick up, even with a baby in them, making it much easier to transport babies around the house.

Infant Carriers/Car Seats

Car seats are the one item that you absolutely can't share among your multiples. In fact, you won't even be able to bring your babies home from the hospital unless you have a car seat for each of them. State laws vary as to how long your children must sit in car seats, but they are mandatory for all infants under twenty pounds.

There are two basic styles of car seats: infant carriers and convertible seats. Infant carriers have two parts: a base that remains affixed to the restraint system in your car, and a detachable carrier seat that cradles the babies. They are only designed for use with babies up to about twenty pounds. Convertible seats remain in the car, meaning that you have to buckle and unbuckle the babies into the seat each time you go for a ride. However, they offer the advantage of longevity, since they can be converted for use with an older baby or toddler.

Even though it means buying multiple versions, purchasing a set of both styles is well worth the investment. The convenience of transporting babies via infant carriers makes the early months much more manageable, but eventually they will outgrow them and you'll need the flexibility of convertible seats.

Swings and Slings

Some babies enjoy passing time in infant swings, and they can be a lifesaver when you have multiples. Don't invest in more than one, however, until you've established that your babies are comfortable in them. Borrow swings, or start off with one, and buy additional swings if it appears your babies appreciate them.

A sling is a comfortable way to carry a baby in a close, bonding manner while keeping your hands free. There are some models designed to accommodate twins, but their use is limited. Some parents find it too awkward or heavy to carry both babies, especially after they reach a certain weight. This is another item that you can borrow or buy singly to experiment with before investing a lot of money to purchase one for each baby.

More Handy Items for Your Multiples

Other products are a must for multiples, but aren't useful until the babies grow up somewhat. These include walkers or exercise saucers, which are useful for babies older than three months. You can wait to buy these until the babies become more mobile. Bath seats keep older babies secure in the tub; it saves time and effort to bathe multiples together, so plan to have one per child.

A play yard is not just handy for keeping multiples in. It's very useful for keeping babies out of situations, as well. Use it to contain pets, to restrict access to off limit areas of the house, or even to surround holiday decorations so that babies can look, but not touch.

Finally, a playpen or play yard is one of the most recommended pieces of equipment for homes with multiples. Playpens are most useful for infants; many are portable and can even be used as temporary or secondary cribs. However, multiple babies soon outgrow the weight limit, just about the time they are needed most! A play yard or designated gated room provides a secure location so that parents can relax and catch their breath. A play yard is a freestanding enclosure, usually composed of sets of interlocking panels. It can be expanded by adding additional panels to accommodate even five, six, or more children. Although it's not needed for infants, down the road it will serve many uses, and bring much peace of mind.

Chapter 11

Adapting Your Lifestyle

There's no doubt that having multiples will change your life forever. But how will they impact your lifestyle, the day-to-day routines of work, play, and home? Will the babies slide right into your family's existing schedule, or do you need to make some changes to accommodate their arrival? As you anticipate some of the ways that twins will impact your relationships and activities, you'll be better equipped to anticipate any necessary adjustments and make a smooth transition into your new lifestyle.

Creating a Workable Budget

Your financial situation will surely be affected. From medical bills to dual college savings plans, the costs of raising simultaneous siblings can be exorbitant. Careful financial planning is crucial to surviving without breaking the bank.

Income Versus Expenses

To establish a workable budget, start with your assets. What income is available for spending? If you're used to being a two-income family, consider the impact of the pregnancy and impending birth on Mom's earning status. Does she stand to lose money due to pregnancy bed rest, childbirth, or maternity leave? Will she return to work after the babies arrive? Will Dad need to take any extended leave?

ESSENTIAL

Some companies offer discounts or incentive programs for families with multiples and it is well worth your time to investigate them. In most cases, you'll be required to write a letter and furnish copies of the babies' birth certificates. For more information, search the Internet for "multiple birth discount program" or check with your local parents of multiples organization.

After evaluating your income, make a list of expense categories, such as housing, utilities, food, transportation, insurance, entertainment, and clothing. Identify categories in three ways: fixed (payment due every month at the same time), flexible (varying in amount), or periodic (paid quarterly or annually). Using past bills and statements, generate an estimate of how much you historically spend on each category.

Now list your anticipated expenses or increases due to multiples: furnishings, equipment, child care, medical bills, diapers, formula (if bottle feeding), clothing, etc. Estimate how much you'll need to spend for each item. It's not an exact science; just a small amount of research will give you enough information to craft a reasonable guess. Compare your income to your expenses. If they're basically equivalent, or if your income exceeds your expenses, you're in good shape. But if you're like most people, your expenses far outweigh your income.

Making Ends Meet

You have two choices: increase your income or reduce your expenses. You can accomplish the first option by taking out loans, by earning a return on investments, or by someone changing jobs or adding a job. It's generally easier and less risky to attempt the second option, reducing expenses.

There are several ways to reduce expenses. Some of them may dwindle naturally due to your lifestyle change after having multiples. For example, you may find that you spend a lot less on entertainment and travel because you don't go out as often while your multiples are young. But in some areas it may require some conscious action to cut back, perhaps by clipping coupons, switching to lower cost services, or cutting out nonessentials.

If the basis of your financial concern is centered around spending on the babies, take heart. There are many strategies for obtaining the items you need at a discount. For starters, there is a tremendous market for used baby equipment, especially among your fellow families with multiples. Network with your local parents of multiples organization to find great buys on used strollers, highchairs, cribs, and everything else you'll need. Thrift stores and consignment shops are also good sources for baby bargains.

In addition, you're likely to be the beneficiary of generous gifts from family and friends. People love to buy for babies, especially when there's more than one. If you are having a baby shower, be politely specific about your needs, and chances are they'll be met.

Working It Out

Unless you've won the lottery or have a money tree growing in the backyard, someone in the family is going to have to generate some income to pay the bills. Since it's going to be a good eighteen years before your multiples are able to earn their keep, that someone is likely to be one or both parents. One of the biggest decisions that parents will have to confront is the issue of working versus staying at home to care for the new arrivals. Basically it boils down to this: give up a paycheck, or pay someone else to care for your babies.

For some families, the choice, one way or the other, is clear. Your financial requirements may demand a dual income to survive. Or perhaps staying at home is the fulfillment of a long-sought dream. But other families face some heavy-duty soul searching and number crunching to reach a solution.

FACT

The Family and Medical Leave Act allows both mothers and fathers to take a total of twelve work weeks of unpaid leave during any twelve-month period. Although you won't earn any money during your leave, it is a particularly welcome benefit for parents of multiples during those busy months with newborns. To find out if you are eligible, visit the U.S. Department of Labor's Web site at *www.dol.gov/esa/whd/fmla/.*

Making the Decision

There are many factors to consider in making the decision, among them career impact, child-care options, parenting philosophy, and expenses. It may be helpful to sit down with your partner and make some notes. Sort out your feelings and discuss any anxieties. Weigh the pros and cons of each option and compare the consequences. Examine the long-term and the short-term benefits of each approach. Both parents should evaluate their earning ability, potential benefits such as health insurance, and their personal goals and desires. Then you'll be able to make a joint decision that will benefit the entire family.

If you are conflicted about this decision, there are some alternative work options that can give you the best of both worlds. Flexible scheduling, job sharing, or working from home are some of the ways that you can generate an income while maximizing your time as a caregiver. If your existing employer isn't willing to explore these options, it may be a good time to consider a career change.

If you decide to stay home and this will be a new role for you, you may be concerned about your changing identity. Rest assured that like any job, although it has its moments of frustration and drudgery, it is also tremendously rewarding. For your twins or more, it's a once-in-a-lifetime opportunity—their lifetime, that is. You can never return to the precious early years of their infancy and babyhood, and they pass by very quickly. Enjoy the opportunity while it lasts.

Child-Care Options

If working full-time appears to be the best option for both parents, you'll need to arrange suitable child care for your multiples. All parents want the best possible care for their children, but there are some inherent challenges in finding quality care for two or more infants. It may require more effort to locate the right situation, so it's best to start your search as soon as you're firm in your decision to work.

In-Home or Center Care

There are several different options for child care, and each approach has distinct advantages and disadvantages. If you can afford it, in-home care is optimal, as your babies remain in a familiar environment and you have a great deal of control over their routines and activities. Nannies and au pairs are two examples of in-home care, which is usually the most expensive style of child care. However, it becomes more economically feasible when you have multiples since you're not paying for each child individually.

Even if you don't require full-time care for your children, consider lining up some assistance anyway. Whether it is a scheduled or occasional babysitter, you'll value the opportunity to leave your twins or more with a trusted helper so that you can work part-time, run errands, spend time with your spouse, or just take a break.

If you seek an outside source of care, such as a daycare center or a sitter who watches children in her own home, you need to make sure that the caregivers adhere to all appropriate licensing and certification requirements. Many states limit the ratio of adults to children, so an individual provider may not be able to accommodate your multiples. Busy daycare facilities may not have sufficient availability for both of your twins or all three of your triplets.

Maintaining Your Marriage

Many parents acknowledge that the experience of having multiples is a true test of their relationship. After the earthquake of multiples rocks your world, there are bound to be some aftershocks, and many times they are felt between husband and wife. Amid the endless cycle of crying, feeding, and diapering babies, it can be very difficult to make your marriage a priority. Remember, however, that sustaining your relationship as a couple is an important part of keeping your family strong. Put your marriage into a long-term perspective and don't get bogged down by the short-term demands of your babies.

Despite the changes that multiples bring to your life, many of your physical and emotional needs will remain the same. Use constructive communication to express your needs and desires. Perhaps you want your husband to show that he appreciates you. Or maybe you'd like your wife to acknowledge your help more often.

In order to make your marriage a priority, you're going to have to invest some time in it, and not just a rushed minute here and there as you hand off baby duties. Schedule time together as you would any other appointment. It could be a lunch date during a workday, or an evening out while a sitter keeps the babies. Then use that time wisely and enjoy each other. Don't turn it into a complaining session where you find fault with one another. Remember why you married each other in the first place!

Dad's Role

New fathers of multiples may feel overlooked when so much attention is heaped on the mother during the pregnancy and the babies after the birth. It's easy to feel lost in the shuffle. In fact, a typical male reaction is to withdraw from the situation. However, this is the time to overcome your instincts and remember that this is not an experience that is only happening to your partner; as the father of multiples, enjoy your chance to equally share in the joys and frustrations of the babies' care.

During the pregnancy, the mother retains most of the physical control of the babies' nurturing and growth. That doesn't exclude fathers as an active participant. Through your support of their mother, you are giving your babies the best possible start in life. Make it your goal to nurture your wife. Prepare healthy snacks for her, bring her a glass of water, and encourage her to rest up as much as possible. If your physician recommends bed rest during the pregnancy, it will likely fall to you to pick up the pieces on the home front, fulfilling the obligations that she would normally carry out.

Emotional Support

In addition to physical support, you play an important emotional role. Worries about coping with pregnancy complications, labor, breastfeeding, and managing infant multiples loom large in the mind of an expectant mother. Hormonal fluctuations and the physical impact of pregnancy on a mother's body intensify her emotions. Your positive and upbeat attitude will go a long way toward reducing stress and dispelling your partner's anxieties. Educate yourself to prepare for the challenges ahead; talk to other fathers about their experiences, read books about multiples (such as this one), and investigate Internet resources (see Appendix A for a list of helpful sites). Going along to doctor appointments and checkups will be a reassuring experience for both of you.

As a dad of twins, you're in good company. Many well-known leaders, actors, writers, and sports figures have fathered multiples. For example, William Shakespeare had fraternal twins. Mohammed Ali is a father of twin daughters, as was Nat King Cole. Actors Mel Gibson, Robert De Niro, and Jimmy Stewart all fathered twins. And George W. Bush once said that raising twin girls was harder than being president!

The good news about being a father of twins or more is that you have the opportunity to be more fully involved in their care than a father of singletons might. You have an important extra set of hands that will be much in demand. The bad news is that you *have* to be fully involved in their care. With extra mouths to feed and bottoms to diaper, there is never a lack of work to be done. Find a niche, a chore that you can master, such as preparing the day's bottles, bathing the babies, or doing the laundry, and then take responsibility for that activity without having to be asked.

Above all, in the midst of the chaos and confusion, help your partner to keep things in perspective. The hectic pace of managing newborn multiples is temporary; life will eventually resume a semblance of normality.

Preparing Siblings

If you already have other children, you may be concerned about how the arrival of twins or more will impact them. There's no way around it; there are some changes in store. It's important to properly prepare them for their new role as big brother or sister of multiples.

Educate and involve your children from the beginning. Introduce them to twinning concepts, and update them on the babies' development throughout the pregnancy. Once the babies arrive, identify specific, age-appropriate ways that they can help their younger siblings. Even toddlers can contribute by fetching supplies!

Meeting Siblings' Needs

As you prepare for your multiples, also consider your child-care needs for your other children. You may have to provide alternative care for them in the event of bed rest or hospitalization during pregnancy. Designate a caregiver in advance, and inform your children of the plans beforehand so that they are familiar and comfortable with the situation. The same goes for their arrangements during delivery. Having a trusted friend or grandparent available to help care for siblings allows you to focus on the newborns.

Your older children may feel displaced or overlooked when the new arrivals come on the scene. Assuage their distress by planning some special surprises that focus attention on them and their importance as "big" brothers or sisters. Stash away some toys or gifts to present at opportune moments, especially items that can keep them quietly occupied when you're busy with the babies. More than gifts, they'll likely crave your time and undivided attention, so make it a priority to preserve cherished routines that provide an opportunity for one-on-one time, such as a morning snuggle, after-school chat, or bedtime story.

ALERT!

You're sure to hear plenty of horror stories about preterm labor, premature babies, breastfeeding nightmares, sleepless nights, and the like. Keep it in perspective. People love to recount their negative experiences; the easy parts don't make for interesting retelling.

Handling Stress

Families experience stress for many reasons, but having multiples generates a unique combination of physical and emotional strain that can push many people to the breaking point. Equipping yourself with coping strategies is one of the best ways to prepare yourself for the challenges ahead, and can help diffuse stress before it builds to a crescendo.

In many cases, the stress begins in pregnancy, with anxiety about medical risks and an unknown future. Don't let your worries cast a negative shadow over your pregnancy experience. Keep a positive outlook. Talk to other multiple birth families about their experiences. You'll notice that, in most cases, everything turned out fine. Everyone survived and is thriving.

If you are a spiritual person, you will likely find great reassurance in practicing your faith. Many families find that prayer and meditation not only calm their anxieties, but also have a positive impact on their well-being—and the babies', as well. Relying on a higher power can carry you through the times when your life seems out of control.

Once the babies are born, the stress continues. Lack of sleep, hormonal fluctuations, and the constant demands of baby care culminate to produce stressed-out parents. It's important to remember that the situation is temporary. "This **two** shall pass" is a favorite mantra of twin parents.

Chapter 12

Complications

Sometimes things go wrong. There are a number of complications associated specifically with multiple birth, as well as an increased risk of other disorders that impact pregnancy. Fortunately, if diagnosed in time, many of these conditions can be remedied before the babies are even born, or shortly after birth.

Twin-to-Twin Transfusion Syndrome

Twin-to-twin transfusion syndrome (TTTS) may sound like a plot from a science fiction movie, but it's an actual phenomenon that can occur during a twin pregnancy. Undetected or untreated, it can have devastating consequences for the babies. However, new treatment options give doctors the ability to correct the situation and offer new hope to parents impacted by the disease.

The effects of TTTS can produce a great deal of variability in the appearance of monozygotic or "identical" twins. The donor twin is usually much smaller and paler, while the recipient twin is larger with a ruddier complexion.

What Is It?

TTTS, also known as feto-fetal transfusion syndrome or stuck twin syndrome, is a disease of the placenta. It doesn't make the mother sick, and its effect on the babies is environmental, not direct. In other words, the babies will begin to develop perfectly normally, but because the placenta they depend on to supply oxygen and nutrition malfunctions, they risk heart failure, brain trauma, and damage to their organs.

The placenta circulates blood and nutrients from the mother to her babies. Within a shared placenta, blood vessels called *chorioangiopagous* vessels may develop, connecting the circulatory systems of both babies via the placenta. This causes an unequal exchange of blood flow between the babies. Essentially, one fetus becomes a donor, pumping blood into the second, recipient fetus. This situation causes problems for both babies, with the donor twin not getting enough blood and the recipient receiving an excess.

The donor twin is at risk for anemia, intrauterine growth retardation, and restricted amniotic fluid (oligohydramnios). While the donor's growth is stunted, the recipient twin grows larger and larger. The extra blood overloads his circulatory system and puts him at risk for heart failure. As he struggles to process the extra blood, his urine production results in an excess of amniotic fluid (polyhydramnios). Eventually, polyhydramnios can trigger the onset of preterm labor and both babies are at risk of being born too early to survive outside the womb.

FACT

As the amount of fluid surrounding the recipient twin increases, the donor twin may be pushed to one side of the uterus. As her fluid levels decrease, she may appear to be stuck to the wall of the womb. Thus, the term "stuck twin syndrome" has been used to describe this condition.

The timing of the disease ultimately determines the prognosis for the babies. It is easier to overcome later in pregnancy, when the simplest solution is to deliver the babies. Although they may face the consequences of a premature birth, they will escape the threat to their survival that exists if they remain in the womb. However, if the onset of TTTS occurs earlier, before the babies are viable, the situation is more dire, although there are treatment options. There are five stages of TTTS:

- **Stage I:** Small amount of fluid in donor baby, large amount in the recipient
- **Stage II:** Symptoms of Stage I, along with undetectable bladder in the donor twin
- **Stage III:** One or both babies will have evidence of poor blood flow
- **Stage IV:** Characterized by hydrops in either baby (a fluid accumulation that signifies heart failure)
- **Stage V:** One or both babies have succumbed

When TTTS is detected in the second trimester, it is usually termed chronic or severe. After twenty-four weeks, it is defined as moderate. When it occurs later in the third trimester, it is labeled mild or acute.

Who Gets It?

Not all twins are at risk for the condition. It only affects a percentage of monozygotic twins, those individuals resulting from one egg. Depending on when the egg splits and implants, monozygotic twins may develop individual placentas or share a single placenta. TTTS only occurs when there is a single, shared placenta.

The term monochorionic describes twins that are joined in a single chorion, the membrane that attaches to a single placenta. Only monochorionic twins are at risk for TTTS because they are the only type whose circulatory systems may connect through the placenta. Although there has been some speculation that two fused placentas could develop a circulatory connection susceptible to TTTS, researchers of the disease confirm that it is simply not feasible.

ALERT!

TTTS only affects monozygotic twins. It occurs in about a third of monochorionic pregnancies, or less than 10 percent of all identical twins. If untreated, it has as much as an 80 percent fetal mortality rate.

How Is It Diagnosed?

One of the reasons that a multiple pregnancy is subjected to closer scrutiny is so TTTS can be detected. Doctors use ultrasound to assess the risk by determining the number of placentas. If there is just one, subsequent ultrasounds will follow the babies' growth and development, as well as the amount of amniotic fluid, to confirm that it remains equalized. If a discrepancy develops, further ultrasound testing may reveal the presence of too much or too little amniotic fluid around each baby, a sure sign that a shared circulatory connection is shunting blood between the babies.

What Can Be Done?

In past times, babies affected by TTTS were doomed. Without ultrasound technology to detect the disorder, it was likely that one or both of the babies would die in utero, or that they would be born too early to survive. Now, not only does sonography enable doctors to diagnose the condition, new treatments allow it to be cured.

Up until very recently, the primary treatment approach was to stave off preterm labor until the babies were viable and could be delivered. This was accomplished by draining the excess fluid surrounding the recipient twin. Amnioreduction, a procedure similar to amniocentesis, was performed at regular intervals to remove fluid from the recipient baby's amnionic sac. While it is generally effective in stabilizing the situation, it carries the same risks as amniocentesis, including infection and miscarriage. It also does not compensate for the damage occurring to the donor twin.

In the 1990s, Dr. Julian DeLia developed an amazing procedure that allows doctors to correct TTTS by using a laser to seal off the connections in the placenta. The procedure is performed while the babies are still in utero, using a fetoscope, a powerful telescope allowing a surgeon to see inside the womb through a tiny incision. A 2004 study confirmed that this procedure, fetoscopic laser coagulation, produces a better outcome for the babies.

Treatment for TTTS depends on how far along you are in your pregnancy, and to which stage the disease has progressed. Fetoscopic laser surgery is available in half a dozen facilities in the United States as well as other locations in Australia and Europe. As studies confirm its success in treating TTTS, it will become more widely available in the next few years. The resources listed in Appendix A include contact information for TTTS support and treatment.

"Mo-Mo" Twins: The Danger of Being Monoamniotic

While TTTS is inflicted upon monochorionic twins, another class of monozygotic twins is subjected to even more dangers. Monochorionic/monoamniotic ("mo-mo") twins share not only a placenta, but an amniotic sac as well. They float together in a single encasement of fluid. They develop this way due to the delayed splitting of the egg, usually about eight days post-fertilization, after a single yolk sac has begun to develop.

FACT

Mo-mo is an extremely rare type of twinning, affecting less than 1 percent of all twin pregnancies. It's also a very dangerous situation, as every time the twins move, they jeopardize each other's survival.

Cord entanglement is the primary risk associated with mo-mo twins. Nearly all will experience some tangling of the umbilical cords as they move around in the womb. Entanglement by itself does not harm the babies. However, if the intertwining results in compression of either cord, the babies' supply of blood and nutrients from the placenta can be cut off, resulting in fetal death. Unfortunately, most of the ensnarling occurs early in pregnancy, when the babies still have plenty of room to move around in the uterine environment. And the longer the cords remain entwined, the greater the risk of damage or death to one or both babies.

How Is It Diagnosed?

Like many other conditions in multiple pregnancy, this type of twinning is detected by ultrasound scan. The presence of same-sex twins and the lack of a dividing membrane could indicate mo-mo twins. Even a thin or vague membrane could be cause for concern; sometimes late twinning can create a membrane that is so thin or full of holes that the babies are able to breach it. Mo-mo twins are often misdiagnosed early in pregnancy. Sometimes a dividing membrane is not visible on ultrasound until the third trimester.

What Can Be Done?

Ultimately, the cure for this condition is to deliver the babies. Parents of mo-mo twins will play a waiting game throughout pregnancy, constantly monitoring the situation until the babies are viable and can be delivered, at some point after twenty-four weeks. While they may suffer the consequences of prematurity, they will no longer be under threat of death in the womb.

Fortunately, cord entanglement usually happens gradually and can be monitored using a Doppler sonogram to measure the blood flow in the umbilical cords. The frequency of scans will depend on your situation; in some cases, constant monitoring requires the mother to be hospitalized for the duration of her pregnancy. Other times, scans will be scheduled at regular intervals, perhaps weekly.

In this situation, delivery by cesarean section is required; even minimal tangling of the cords produces a risk of cord prolapse, a serious condition where the cord of the second baby is extruded as the first baby is delivered. The risks are so high that doctors aren't willing to attempt a vaginal delivery.

The survival rate for mo-mo babies is estimated at about 60 percent. However, their odds are improving as doctors experiment with new treatments to sustain the pregnancy, including a drug called Sulindac that reduces the amount of amniotic fluid, restricting the babies' movement, and minimizing chances of entanglement.

Conjoined Twinning

Conjoined, or Siamese, twins are another type of monozygotic twins that occur due to late splitting of the fertilized egg. Conjoined twinning is extremely rare, occurring in only 1 in 100,000 births. The majority of conjoined twins are female, although no one is exactly sure why that is. Every set of conjoined twins has a unique connection, but about three-quarters of conjoined twins are connected at the torso.

Generally, conjoined twins result if the split is delayed more than twelve days post-fertilization; the later the split, the more tissue and organ function is shared. The degree of conjoinedness determines the outlook for the babies; few sets are able to survive without surgical separation. Many do not even survive in the womb—more than half are stillborn.

Surgical separation of conjoined twins attracts much media attention, but unfortunately, many conjoined twins are not candidates for surgery. Babies who share major organ function cannot survive separately, putting parents in the unthinkable position of having to sacrifice one child for the survival of the other. Advances in medical technology are giving parents more hope, however, as doctors gain more expertise in the treatment of this unique kind of twinning.

Conjoined twins are sometimes known as Siamese twins, a reference to Chang and Eng Bunker, the first set of conjoined twins to gain world renown. Born in Siam in the early 1800s, they traveled the world as circus performers before settling down and marrying sisters in North Carolina.

High Blood Pressure (Hypertension)

While many complications in multiple pregnancy put the babies at risk, one in particular jeopardizes the mother. Mothers of multiples are particularly susceptible to a group of diseases associated with elevated blood pressure.

Pregnancy Induced Hypertension (PIH)

Increased blood pressure—generally measured as higher than 140 over 90—is common in mothers of multiples. It is treated by reducing activity, even to the point of bed rest, and sometimes with medication. Generally, hypertension associated with pregnancy will dissipate as soon as the babies are born, but these women may be at risk for high blood pressure later in life, especially in subsequent pregnancies.

Preeclampsia/Toxemia

A more serious condition affecting mothers of multiples is preeclampsia, also known as toxemia. Less than 10 percent of singleton pregnancies are impacted by preeclampsia, but it is much more common in mothers of multiples. About one in three women expecting twins, triplets, or more will suffer from it during pregnancy. While it is often confused with hypertension, two other symptoms must be present in order for a diagnosis of preeclampsia to be confirmed: edema and elevated protein in the urine.

The elevation in blood pressure inflicts damage to small capillaries, which leak fluid into surrounding tissue and cause edema, or swelling. Most pregnant women experience some degree of swelling, especially in the later months of pregnancy, but edema is characterized by a sudden onset that persists throughout the day. In addition to edema, preeclampsia is characterized by proteinuria, the presence of significant amounts of protein in the urine (this signifies kidney malfunction). Preeclampsia can precede a more serious condition, eclampsia, which can lead to seizures, stroke, kidney failure, a ruptured liver, and problems with blood clotting.

There is evidence to suggest that a diet rich in calcium and omega-3 fatty acids in the form of fish oil can reduce the incidence of preeclampsia in pregnancy. You should discuss the possible benefits of this with your health-care provider before taking any dietary supplements.

Preeclampsia usually affects women in the latter half of pregnancy, but the longer a woman combats it, the greater the potential for complications. There is no cure for the condition; the only remedy is to deliver the babies. Medical caregivers have to weigh the deterioration of the mother's state against the babies' outlook for survival if born early.

Notify your doctor immediately if you experience the symptoms of preeclampsia, including sudden swelling in the hands or face, rapid weight gain, blurred vision, seeing spots, intense headache, or abdominal pain. Generally, at the first sign of symptoms, you'll be advised to restrict your activity and may even be assigned to bed rest. Sometimes medications may be administered, such as magnesium sulfate, a drug commonly used to treat preterm labor that also temporarily lowers blood pressure.

HELLP Syndrome

Fifteen percent of women with preeclampsia will develop HELLP syndrome, an abbreviation for hemolysis, elevated liver enzymes, and low platelets. This condition is due to disturbance of the liver's normal function, and mothers with HELLP can die from a ruptured liver if they are not treated. Sometimes the syndrome progresses before the symptoms of preeclampsia are identified, because women can develop HELLP in the absence of hypertension, edema, and protein in the urine. Be sure to report any unusual symptoms to your doctor, such as abdominal pain on the right side, fatigue, nausea, vomiting, or headache. These can be signs of HELLP syndrome.

Gestational Diabetes

Gestational diabetes in pregnancy is not the same as a diagnosis of diabetes outside of pregnancy. Although the disorder is similar—the inability of the body to process glucose (sugar) in the blood—the cause is directly related to pregnancy, and the condition should disappear after delivery. However, it is important to get treatment, because when glucose backs up in the bloodstream, it can damage the mother's organs, and possibly the babies as well.

Gestational diabetes occurs two to three times more often in multiple pregnancy than in singleton pregnancies. The increase is likely due to the additional hormones produced when there are extra babies; hormones can interfere with the body's ability to process the insulin produced by the pancreas.

ESSENTIAL

Most health-care providers routinely screen for gestational diabetes during pregnancy. A glucose challenge test is usually administered toward the end of the second trimester or early in the third.

If you are diagnosed with gestational diabetes during your pregnancy with multiples, you will need to alter your diet. In some cases, gestational diabetes may be controlled with lifestyle and nutrition management, but if your case does not respond, you may require injections of insulin for the duration of your pregnancy. Fortunately, gestational diabetes has little effect on the babies, although they may be at risk of contracting diabetes later in life.

Placenta Problems

The placenta plays a vital role in pregnancy, delivering nutrients and oxygen to the babies and removing their waste. In a multiple pregnancy, each baby may have his own placenta, or two babies may share a single placenta. Either way, if something goes wrong, the babies' survival is at stake.

Placenta Previa

When the placenta implants low in the uterus, covering the cervical opening, it's called placenta previa. The chances of this happening are increased when a uterus has to accommodate two or more placentas. While placenta previa does not pose a risk to the babies' development, it may cause vaginal bleeding toward the conclusion of the pregnancy, as the cervix begins to dilate and open. Bed rest may help the bleeding subside by decreasing the amount of pressure on the placenta. In extreme cases, the mother may require a blood transfusion to prevent excess blood loss. Usually she will have to deliver the babies via cesarean section.

Abruptio Placentae

Sometimes the placenta begins to detach prematurely from the wall of the uterus, a condition called abruptio placentae. While it can be caused by trauma to the abdominal region, it can also be instigated by other conditions that are common in a multiple pregnancy, such as high blood pressure. The detachment may be mild and partial, happening slowly over time, or complete and sudden. Pain and bleeding usually accompanies complete abruption; this requires immediate delivery of the babies by c-section. In more mild cases, doctors will closely monitor the pregnancy to determine the best option for the babies, weighing the consequences of early delivery. Bed rest may be recommended.

Placental abruptions are three times more common in a multiple pregnancy due to the increased stretching of the uterus as it expands to accommodate the extra babies.

Hemorrhage

Mothers of multiples have an increased risk of hemorrhage, or uncontrolled bleeding, during their pregnancy or following delivery. Several factors contribute to the risk:

- A uterus that is stretched and strained by accommodating additional babies
- A greater portion of the surface area of the uterus covered by placental tissue
- Increased chance of undergoing cesarean section

Usually, the only consequence is heavier postpartum bleeding following delivery, but occasionally severe, uncontrolled bleeding puts the mother's health at risk.

ALERT!

If postpartum bleeding is so heavy that you soak through a sanitary pad in less than an hour, seek medical attention. Additional signs of hemorrhage include bright red bleeding that lingers a week after delivery, vaginal discharge with a foul odor, or discharge that includes blood clots larger than an inch in diameter.

Intrauterine Growth Restriction (IUGR)

Multiples are particularly at risk for intrauterine growth restriction (IUGR), also known as intrauterine growth retardation. Essentially, this very wordy terminology is used to describe a small baby, a baby that is not growing at a "normal" rate according to standardized charts. Babies with IUGR are identified when they are below the tenth percentile on growth charts. IUGR occurs in more than a quarter of twin pregnancies, much more often than in the general population of singleton births, where the occurrence is only 6 percent.

What Causes It?

IUGR can occur as a result of other conditions particular to a multiple birth, such as TTTS, preeclampsia, or a shared placenta. But sometimes just the fact that there is more than one baby competing for resources in the womb causes the restriction in growth. IUGR is the second leading cause of death in infants.

What's the difference between IUGR, SGA, and LBW?
IUGR refers to a baby who has not reached his growth potential because of some medical problem. An SGA (small for gestational age) baby is simply a small baby, growing to his full potential. LBW (low birth weight) is the term used to describe babies after birth, while IUGR and SGA refer to babies while they're still in the womb.

IUGR is defined in three ways:

- **Symmetric IUGR:** The baby's weight, head circumference, and abdominal circumference are all below the tenth percentile; usually attributable to an abnormality or infection.
- **Asymmetric IUGR:** The baby's weight is below the tenth percentile, but the head circumference and body length measure greater than the tenth percentile. It is usually caused by severe placental insufficiency.
- **Combined type IUGR:** The baby may have skeletal shortening and some reduction of soft tissue mass.

IUGR can impact one or all of the babies in a multiple pregnancy. When only one baby is affected, it is sometimes referred to as growth discordance.

What Can Be Done?

IUGR puts babies at risk for stillbirth and neonatal death. Often, the only option for treatment is to deliver the affected baby, or babies. They will be impacted by the usual complications associated with preterm birth, but can be treated for them. The effects of IUGR can follow the babies, even after birth. They're at risk for many long-term neurological and behavioral handicaps that may not surface until many years later. They are often hypoglycemic, and have weak muscle tone and poor circulation. Thirty percent of babies who succumb to SIDS (sudden infant death syndrome) had IUGR.

You can take some steps toward preventing IUGR from impacting your babies. Maternal nutrition is crucial. Eating healthy foods, and plenty of them, provides the energy that your babies need to grow adequately. Maternal tobacco use is a leading cause of IUGR, so it goes without saying that you should stay away from cigarettes. Finally, getting plenty of rest can also help. When you rest, nutrients will pass more easily to the babies, who utilize every calorie to grow and develop. While you can't absolutely prevent IUGR in a multiple pregnancy, there is no doubt that taking tiptop care of yourself is the best way to protect your babies.

Chapter 13

Bed Rest

One of the greatest ironies of multiple birth is that you spend most of your pregnancy trying to avoid bed rest, but once the babies arrive you crave it! Some form of bed rest is a reality for the majority of mothers of multiples during their pregnancy. It can be an important tool in keeping the developing babies healthy and preventing preterm labor. In the event that your doctor recommends bed rest, it's important to understand the ramifications of your situation.

What Bed Rest Accomplishes

Historically, bed rest has been a common treatment for a variety of pregnancy ailments. With fewer side effects than drugs, it can prevent or diminish many problems that would otherwise result in the loss of one or all of the babies. When you're carrying multiples, the goal is to keep them in your womb as long as possible in order to ensure optimal health and development. Usually, women carrying higher order multiples have a greater chance of going on bed rest, have to stay on bed rest for a longer period of time, and have to endure a stricter regimen of bed rest than mothers of singletons.

As the pregnancy progresses, the combined weight of the babies strains the cervix. Gravity increases the pressure. Alleviating the pull of gravity and the pressure on the cervix can help prolong the pregnancy. That can be accomplished by staying off your feet and lying horizontally in bed.

There is much dissension among the medical community as to whether bed rest should be routinely prescribed in multiple pregnancy. Some physicians argue that preventative bed rest should be mandatory for moms of multiples. At one time, bed rest at twenty-eight weeks was the standard for moms of multiples. Fortunately, that's not the case now. Most doctors acknowledge the emotional and psychological toll on the family of a pregnant woman, as well as potential physical deterioration for the mother.

FACT

About 20 percent of pregnancies require bed rest, or about 700,000 women per year. However, it's much more likely in a multiple pregnancy. A 1992 survey from the National Organization of Mothers of Twins Clubs found that it's a factor in 70 percent of multiple pregnancies.

Blood Pressure Benefits

Another common problem in multiple pregnancy is hypertension, or high blood pressure. It can be a symptom of preeclampsia, a serious disorder that, if left untreated, can be fatal for the mother and the babies. (See Chapter 12.) Bed rest can be very effective in lowering blood pressure in pregnancy by taking the pressure of the uterus off the vena cava, a large vein that runs along the right side of the body. Usually mothers who are undergoing bed rest to reduce their blood pressure are advised to lie on their left side to improve circulation.

Placating the Placenta

Dizygotic or multizygotic multiples each have their own placenta, maximizing the surface area of the uterus that is covered by placental matter. This increases the chances of complications, including placenta previa, a condition that occurs when the placenta covers the cervix. The resulting hemorrhage can be dangerous for the mother and impede development of the babies. Bed rest and reduced activity can help diminish the bleeding.

Bed rest also allows more blood and oxygen to flow to the placenta(s), enhancing the growth of the babies. If you're experiencing complications such as preterm labor or placenta previa and your babies will likely be delivered early, a period of bed rest accompanied by treatment with steroids may give them a developmental boost.

Good for Mom

Although bed rest is usually prescribed to benefit the babies, it can be just as beneficial to the mother's well-being. A multiple pregnancy places a tremendous strain on the mother's organs, which work overtime to keep up with the demands of nurturing multiple fetuses. Sometimes rest and relaxation in bed are required to minimize a mother's activity and give her body a break. Often bed rest becomes a last resort for women who can't seem to slow down otherwise.

Be wary if your doctor routinely prescribes bed rest at a particular point in the pregnancy without regard for your individual circumstances. Except in the case of extreme higher order multiples, bed rest should not be mandated without specific conditions that necessitate it.

What to Expect

Every expectant mother of multiples should be aware of the possibility of bed rest during her pregnancy. Although there are plenty of women, especially mothers of twins, who never have a reason to go on bed rest during their pregnancy, you should still be prepared for the eventuality. Awareness and preparation will make the experience much more manageable if it does happen.

Finding Yourself in Bed

Often confinement comes unexpectedly. Perhaps you visited your doctor for a routine checkup and were ordered to bed. Or, you rushed to the hospital with symptoms of preterm labor and were admitted. Once you're assigned to bed, it may be too late to make arrangements and you'll have to scramble to provide coverage for work, family, and other commitments. Usually bed rest becomes a reality later in the pregnancy, but don't assume it only happens in the third trimester. Many mothers of multiples may experience bed rest in the second, or even first, trimester.

Bed rest may be a temporary measure to stabilize a condition, or it may be prescribed for the duration of your pregnancy. The level of confinement may be adjusted as your condition changes. Your restrictions may even be lifted if you surpass the crucial number of gestational weeks and are able to deliver full-term babies.

Bed Rest for Preterm Labor

If you are experiencing preterm labor, your rest may be combined with uterine monitoring to detect contractions. You may also be given medication to reduce contractions and/or accelerate the babies' development.

The evidence is mixed as to whether monitoring is an effective tool for preventing premature birth. Some feel that it is useful in identifying patterns of contractions, while others argue that it causes needless inconvenience and worrying over false alarms.

It's important to fully understand what your doctor expects of you, so that you can comply with the orders. Ask questions to clarify anything you're unsure about. Rebelling against your doctor's advice only endangers your babies, or even your own health. Don't be a martyr. Pushing the limits at home may result in bed rest at the hospital where your doctors can enforce the limitations.

Lying Low

Lying around isn't exactly a bed of roses. Being inactive for an extended period of time can have a negative impact on your body. Weight loss, weakened muscle tone, loss of muscle mass, bone deterioration, and blood clots are all common consequences of bed rest. The general weakness that results may hinder your recovery after delivery and leave you ill-equipped to care for the babies when they arrive.

The psychological toll of bed rest is also a factor to consider. Feelings of anxiety, frustration, and depression are common. Boredom is rampant. Isolation from family, friends, and the workplace only increases the emotional distress. Because a mother's emotional state has a great bearing on her physical well-being, these feelings must be acknowledged and dealt with as conscientiously as her medical condition.

Partial Versus Full Bed Rest

There are various levels of bed rest. Your condition will determine which type is most beneficial to your babies. Recommendations for your situation may vary throughout your pregnancy, depending on your health and the status of the babies.

Often the first stage is decreased or reduced activity. Your doctor may recommend this regardless of your condition, simply to give your body a chance to rest from its work of nurturing multiple babies. Or you may voluntarily cut back on your schedule as your pregnancy progresses and you start feeling more tired or out of sorts. You'll probably be advised to avoid heavy lifting, strenuous exercise, or anything that causes you to exert yourself. This is a time to slow down and take it easy. Spend some time each day with your feet up, or fit a nap into your daily schedule.

Partial Bed Rest

The least restrictive form of actual bed rest is partial bed rest, also called modified or moderate bed rest. The amount of time spent lying down can vary widely. You may be advised to spend a certain number of hours in bed each day or, conversely, you may be allotted a specified amount of time out of bed. Every individual's circumstance is unique; some women are able to continue working and running the household, but most will need to make adjustments to their lifestyle. Your doctor will advise you as to your exact limitations.

Be sure you check with your doctor about allowable activities when you're out of bed. They may be restricted to basic necessities, such as bathing or eating. Other situations may permit short errands and quiet activity around the house. Depending on your condition, you may need to spend the majority of your lying-down time on your left side. If you prefer, you may be able to fulfill this type of bed rest on a couch during daytime hours, rather than a bed, so that you can be more accessible to the household.

ALERT!

Because partial or modified bed rest leaves you with a lot of freedom to control your activity, it's important that you not overdo it. Ask your doctor for explicit instructions as to what is allowed or discouraged.

Complete Bed Rest

Complete bed rest is the strictest level. You'll be required to remain in bed twenty-four hours a day. (If you're lucky, you'll be allowed to get up to use the restroom.) Spending all your time in bed can be a grueling experience. Not only are you prevented from caring for your family, but you will require assistance for your own basic needs. It is likely that you will have to give up work for the time being, unless your job is such that you can work exclusively via phone or laptop computer. Even that may prove difficult if your condition necessitates that you lie in a particular position. Visits to the doctor for checkups are the only respite from this type of bed rest, and even those may be restricted.

Know Why You're in Bed

Whichever level of bed rest that you are assigned, be sure that you understand the reason behind it, and the goal or outcome. Are you trying to maintain your blood pressure? Minimize contractions? If you feel that your doctor is being overly cautious in prescribing bed rest, discuss your concerns. You may be able to negotiate a compromise that satisfies your doctor's conditions but still allows you freedom to do the things you want to do.

Hospitalization for Bed Rest

In extreme situations, you may find yourself confined to bed in the hospital. Sometimes this occurs at the onset of symptoms, before even needing home bed rest. Other times, it is the final result of a bed rest trial at home that simply isn't working. While a period of hospitalization may be stressful and inconvenient, there are also some advantages to being cared for in a professional medical setting.

It's Not All Bad

Being admitted to the hospital during your pregnancy with multiples can be terrifying. It may feel like a prison sentence. You'll likely feel a disturbing loss of control over your life, anxiety about the outcome of your pregnancy, and a fair amount of panic about the responsibilities you've left undone at home or work.

On the other hand, being admitted to the hospital can be reassuring. You can turn over responsibility for your babies' health to professionals. It is comforting to know that you are in the best possible place if anything goes wrong. If you've been on bed rest at home, it may be a relief to have caregivers available to attend to your needs, such as bringing meals or helping you use the toilet. With external circumstances out of your control, you can just lie back (or however you're instructed to lie!), relax, and focus on nurturing the babies inside you.

You'll need to inform your place of employment about your hospital confinement as soon as possible. Depending on your job situation, your absence may be covered by maternity leave, disability leave, or sick leave. Be upfront and honest with your employer about your situation. Pass along any information you have from the doctors as to the timeline of your confinement.

Housekeeping Details

In most cases, you won't have a lot of time to plan for hospitalization. You'll have to rely on your partner, friends, or relatives to cover the details you've left behind until you can make arrangements. Ask someone to bring some things from home that will help make your stay more comfortable:

- Address book or telephone directory
- Loose-fitting, comfortable maternity clothes for daytime
- Loose-fitting, comfortable pajamas for nighttime
- Slippers or socks
- Comfort items from your bed at home, such as a pillow and blanket
- Toiletries and hair care items
- Reading material
- Entertainment, such as books, magazines, puzzles, or crafts
- Pictures from home that make you happy
- CD player with earphones, for listening to calming music or audio books

If you have other children at home, you'll have to arrange for their care in your absence. If the designated caregiver is your spouse, this can be a difficult position for both parents. Fathers may feel torn between their obligations at home and their desire to comfort their wife in the hospital. There may be financial concerns if both parents have to miss work due to the hospitalization.

Surviving Off Your Feet

For the sake of your babies, you have to make the best of bed rest in order to endure it. There are many ways to make the experience more tolerable as you pass the time. It can even be a productive and enjoyable time as you await the arrival of your babies.

Attitude Adjustment

With your physical self temporarily out of commission, you'll have to rely on your mental abilities to gain control of your situation. Your attitude toward your situation can make a huge difference in how you tolerate it. Stress, frustration, and anxiety only serve to make physical problems worse. Adjust your mindset by accepting your circumstances and acknowledging that this temporary confinement will provide the best possible start in life for your precious babies.

Put your situation in perspective. Remember, this is temporary. No one remains pregnant forever. Eventually, the babies will be born and you'll be back on your feet. It may seem unbelievable now, but there will come a day when you'll wish for a few hours alone in bed!

FACT

Prayer, meditation, and relaxation techniques will help you cope with the anxiety and worry. Fill your mind with peaceful, positive images. Play pleasant background music, read lighthearted material, or watch funny movies.

Finally, view your bed rest as an assignment, or a goal, that can be accomplished one step at a time. Get through just one hour at a time, and eventually the hours become days, and the days become weeks. Every extra moment that you give your babies in the womb is beneficial to their development.

Creating a Restful Environment

Once you have your mindset in the right perspective, enlist some help in setting up your "work station"—the place where you'll perform the work of surviving bed rest. Designate a spot in the house where you can position all your supplies within arm's reach. You'll want plenty of healthy snacks and water on hand. Books, magazines, and craft projects help pass the time, if you can concentrate on them. Electronic equipment such as a telephone and remotes to operate a television or DVD player should be easily accessible.

A cooler is a very handy accessory next to your bed. Keep it stocked with nutritious snacks and drinks. Even though your body is not physically active, you need to keep your calorie and fluid intake high.

Creating structure within your day will make the time pass faster. Stick with a routine similar to your normal daily schedule. Get cleaned up and dressed every morning. Brush your hair and put on makeup. Even though you're not going out, you might be welcoming visitors and you'll feel better physically if you look presentable. Wear comfortable maternity clothes, not ratty pajamas. Eat meals and snacks at regularly scheduled times; it will give you something to look forward to! Open the blinds or windows to let the sunshine in each morning and close them when it's dark to signal your body that it's nighttime and time to sleep.

Bed rest is not intended to be one long series of naps. Ask your doctor to define how much sleep you should be getting, and try to keep yourself "active" the rest of the day. Talk to your doctor about any exercise that is safe for you to do in bed or, if you're on modified bed rest, appropriate exercise when you're out of bed. While you don't want to do any activity that would jeopardize your condition, there may be some allowable exercises that will help prevent muscle loss.

Staying Involved

Find ways that you can participate in your family's lifestyle, or a way that you can contribute to chores. For example, you may be able to fold laundry, help children with their homework, research recipes for meals, pay bills online, or even shop for groceries via the Internet. Undertaking a responsibility will give you a sense of purpose and ease your frustration about not being able to care for your household in the normal manner.

Bed rest may cause you to miss out on some of the milestones of pregnancy: your baby shower, shopping for baby supplies, and childbirth education class. If you weren't able to accomplish these earlier in your pregnancy, you may still be able to experience them. It just takes a bit of creative planning. Find out if your childbirth educator can provide a videotape about labor and delivery that you can watch at home. Contact the local mothers of multiples club to find out what educational resources they can provide from their lending library. If you can tolerate the stimulation, you can even preside over a baby shower in your bedroom; you'll just have to ask your guests to bring the party to you!

Finally, use your time wisely. Enjoy the relative peace and quiet that precedes the addition of multiples to a family. Bond with your babies before they're born. You can read to them and sing to them; studies have proven that babies hear voices from inside the womb. Compose a letter for each baby to be given to them at a later date. Organize your family's photos into albums or scrapbooks. Start preparing baby books for each of the babies. If you have sewing or craft skills, create a gift for each baby, such as a crocheted blanket or hat.

Although bed rest adds a frustrating and anxious element to a multiple pregnancy, it can be an important preservation tool for the babies. You'll all make it through just fine if you employ a positive outlook, rely on plenty of outside help, and comply with your doctor's orders.

Chapter 14

Preterm Labor

From the moment you found out you were having multiples, you were likely warned about the risks of preterm labor. It's a problem that affects more than half of twin pregnancies and nearly all higher order multiples. While not every mother-to-be will experience the symptoms of preterm labor, it's very important for everyone to understand the signs in order to get effective help in the event it occurs.

Why Preterm Labor Is a Concern

Preterm labor, or the onset of cervical dilation before a baby is considered full term, is a major source of concern because it can lead to premature delivery. The fact that preterm labor is more prevalent in multiple pregnancy makes it a focus of concern for any expectant mother of twins or more. It's important to look at the true definition of preterm labor in context. Preterm labor is defined as labor that begins before a baby is thirty-seven weeks old. A normal singleton gestation is usually considered to last forty weeks. However, opinions vary on the optimal gestation for multiples. Some define full term as thirty-eight weeks for twins, and thirty-six weeks for higher order multiples. (There is even some evidence to indicate that carrying babies past thirty-eight weeks in a multiple pregnancy can pose risks to the mother's health.)

ESSENTIAL

Mothers of twins are two and one-half times more likely to experience preterm labor than a singleton mother. For higher order multiples, the chances are even higher. However, preterm labor doesn't always result in disaster. Learning about the reality of preterm labor and premature birth should be a lesson in preparation and prevention, not a source of alarm and worry.

So when you see the claims about the high percentage of multiple pregnancies that encounter preterm labor, realize that these cases occur over a vast period of time during the nine months of pregnancy. It may occur as early as the second trimester, with severe consequences, or relatively late in the pregnancy—up to thirty-seven weeks—producing full-term, completely healthy babies.

However, the dangers can't be denied. Preterm labor can lead to premature birth. Despite amazing advances in medical technology, babies born too early simply can't survive outside the womb. You'll find more details about the impact of prematurity in Chapter 17. The simple fact is that preterm birth is the leading cause of neonatal death, and preemies who do survive may face a lifetime of medical problems.

Medical providers focus heavily on raising awareness about preterm labor because, if caught in time, it can be stopped or delayed. Heightened awareness about the risks may prompt a mother to take action and get medical attention sooner rather than later. While it's not always possible to halt preterm labor, in some cases quick medical reaction can increase the chances of success.

Causes of Preterm Labor

The causes of preterm labor are varied and not always identifiable. Certainly if the exact cause was known, treatment to prevent it would be developed. In a normal pregnancy, hormones signal the body to go into labor when the baby is ready to be born. In order for labor to occur, two things must happen:

- Regular coordinated contractions of the uterus
- Changes in the cervix, including effacement (thinning) and dilation (opening)

With preterm labor, something triggers a physiological miscommunication, and the labor process begins too early. In a multiple pregnancy, any number of factors can ignite the process.

Physical Causes

There are several physical factors that contribute to the onset of preterm labor. One factor that can trigger the uterus to begin contracting is its size. Clearly, that's one reason why mothers of multiples are more prone to preterm labor. When a uterus contains more than one baby, it is going to expand to a greater size more quickly! But if that was the only trigger for preterm labor, then all mothers of twins or more would delivery early, and that's certainly not the case.

While we tend to think of a mother's womb as a tender and nurturing place, some factors can make it irritable or hostile. In response, it begins to contract, resulting in the onset of preterm labor. Some experts believe that a lack of circulation is a leading cause. Physical exertion, and even simply standing upright, causes the uterus to settle on top of the arteries and veins that exist along the pelvis. The increasing weight of the babies compresses the arteries, reducing blood flow and hampering circulation. In response, the uterus begins to contract in an effort to release the pressure and restore circulation. This problem is obviously worsened by the added weight of multiple babies, but it can also be influenced by the shape of the uterus.

FACT

The daughters of women who took DES during their pregnancy are particularly plagued by the uterine deformities that can cause preterm labor. DES (diethylstilbestrol) was a drug given to women in the middle of the twentieth century to prevent miscarriage, but was found to cause birth defects.

Infection can also cause a response from the uterus. Expectant mothers of multiples need to be especially wary of infections of their genitals and urological system. Report any signs of kidney or urinary tract infections to your doctor.

The uterus isn't the only culprit in the battle against preterm labor. Remember, the cervix plays an equally important role in the labor process. The cervix is the opening between the uterus and the vagina, and if it malfunctions by starting its job too early, it can be the cause of preterm labor. During pregnancy, it should remain tightly closed, keeping the babies in and everything else out! But sometimes it starts the process of thinning out and opening up too early. This is referred to as an incompetent cervix, and although it can happen to any woman, the added strain of a multiple pregnancy can contribute to the condition. The good news is that an incompetent cervix can be treated. Unfortunately, however, it often isn't discovered until it's too late to prevent delivery.

The womb is a complicated system. Sometimes, even though the uterus and cervix behave appropriately, other malfunctions may produce the onset of labor. Weakened amniotic membranes, problems with the placenta, or the presence of fibroids are a few of the more common conditions. In addition, one or all of the babies may be the source of the mixed signals.

Congenital defects, more common in multiples than singletons, often trigger an early onset of labor.

Don't let the scary statistics convince you that preterm labor is in your future. For a good proportion of twin pregnancies, it's not an issue at all. Be prepared and informed, but don't adopt a negative mindset by assuming that it will happen to you.

Environmental Causes

In addition to the numerous physical conditions that exist, there are several environmental impacts that can trigger preterm labor. Some of them are modifiable or avoidable, while others are simply inherent risks of heredity or lifestyle. Sometimes these factors are intensified in a multiple pregnancy.

Preterm labor may occur as a result of an accident that causes trauma to the mother's abdomen. An auto accident or a fall down the stairs is always unfortunate, but during pregnancy such an incident can have a devastating impact on the babies. While you can't prevent accidents, you can minimize your risk by being extra cautious during pregnancy and avoiding dangerous situations.

Opinions are mixed on whether stress causes preterm labor, but emotional upheaval has been proven to have a negative impact on pregnancy. Some theorize that emotional strain increases the level of corticotropin-releasing hormone (CRH), which can prompt the release of prostaglandin, ultimately triggering contractions. At any rate, studies clearly show a connection between stressed-out mothers and low-birth-weight babies. While reducing stress may not prevent preterm labor, it can enhance your babies' development, improving their odds in the event they do arrive ahead of schedule.

Many environmental risk factors associated with lifestyle can be modified or alleviated, especially if the mother makes changes before becoming pregnant. Women who are either overweight or underweight have an elevated risk of experiencing preterm labor, so good nutrition before conception is important. Smoking, drinking alcohol, and using illegal drugs all vastly increase the levels of risk, not just of preterm labor but of a host of other problems and complications.

Although it may cause contractions, sexual intercourse is not usually a cause of preterm labor. Unless your medical provider advises you to refrain from sex, don't let fear of preterm labor keep you from intimacy.

Ways to Reduce Your Risk

So you accept the fact that there's a chance that your twins, triplets, or more could come early. Is there anything you can do to improve your odds? Although no one can eliminate the risk, there are some things that you can do—or not do—to take control of your pregnancy.

What Not to Do

The duration of pregnancy is less than a year, and you want it to last as long as possible to ensure the health of your babies. So during those months while you're expecting, take time off from any activities that might increase your risk of preterm labor. Certainly any strenuous or dangerous sports are out of the question. But even moderate activity can aggravate the conditions that prompt preterm labor when you're carrying two or more. Use good judgment about your behavior and avoid exertion.

As you go further along in your pregnancy, avoid lifting anything heavy. You probably won't mind being excused from hefting around the vacuum cleaner or toting packages, but this can be a difficult assignment if you have other children, especially young toddlers who want to be held or carried. When you do have to lift something, be sure to use proper posture to avoid strain. Keep your cool in the summertime, when heat and humidity run rampant. The risk of preterm labor increases with the temperature since your body is more likely to be stressed when it is overheated.

What to Do

Diet and nutrition can have a big impact on the outcome of your pregnancy. While there's no magic menu that will keep you out of harm's way, you can actively contribute to your babies' health by eating healthfully and amply. Sufficient calorie intake helps your babies grow and develop, preventing intrauterine growth retardation (IUGR) and low birth weight. In the event that they are born early, they'll stand a much better chance of survival.

Drink plenty of water. The link between dehydration and contractions is clear and unmistakable. Dehydration causes contractions. Rehydration can sometimes stop them. Drink your fill of water every day to keep the contractions at bay.

Give your body the rest it needs. In a multiple pregnancy, gravity is working against you. Taking time off your feet alleviates pressure on your pelvis. Follow your provider's guidelines for rest. Aside from physically resting, it's also important to relax mentally. Emotional stress can aggravate preterm labor. When you get angry or upset, your hormones go into high gear, elevating your blood pressure and heart rate. That diverts circulation from your uterus, which may start contracting in response.

ALERT!

Take care of your teeth. Women with gum disease are seven times more likely to experience preterm labor because of a raised risk of infection.

Finally, education and awareness are two of your strongest weapons against preterm labor. Understand the signs so that you can recognize them if they happen to you. Stay in close contact with your medical provider. Attend all scheduled prenatal visits. Follow recommendations and don't push the envelope if you are assigned limitations. Report any suspicious symptoms, even if it's just a feeling that something's not quite right.

Signs of Preterm Labor

How will you know if preterm labor starts during your pregnancy with multiples? There are some clues, but they might not be obvious until it's too late to stop a delivery: That's why it is so vitally important to know the signals, and to contact your medical provider as soon as you suspect something.

Contractions

Sometimes preterm labor is silent. Many women don't realize that their body is undermining their pregnancy until it's too late—or rather, too early for their premature babies. You won't feel an incompetent cervix dilating or effacing. You may not even feel contractions, especially if you've never been pregnant before.

The uterus contracts throughout pregnancy. These irregular, "practice" contractions are called Braxton-Hicks contractions and they can start as early as the second trimester. As the body readies for labor and delivery, however, the timing, regularity, and intensity of the contractions will increase.

It is the pattern and frequency of the contractions that can signal that labor is imminent. Occasional or irregular contractions are normal. Recurring contractions at a rate of more than four per hour are cause for concern and require further monitoring.

Know Your Body

Women experience contractions in different ways; they may produce a sensation of pain, hardening, pressure, heaviness, tightening, or cramping. They may be felt in the abdomen, pelvis, and lower back, or even the upper thighs. You'll have to spend some time getting to know your body to understand how the contractions will be manifested in your multiple pregnancy. The best way to tune into contractions is to lie quietly on your left side. Put your hands on your belly. You may feel protruding baby parts, such as a head, elbow, or rear end. These will feel hard and bumpy; feel for a softer spot so that you can feel your uterus and not the movement of the babies. At rest, your uterus will feel soft and fleshy, but when contracted, it will feel tight and hard, like a flexed muscle.

Suspicious Signs

The following symptoms and situations should be reported to your caregiver:

- More than four or five contractions per hour
- Rhythmic or persistent pelvic pressure
- Cramps, similar to menstrual cramping
- Backache

ALERT!

Don't ignore the signs. Your body may be trying to cue you that something is wrong. A prompt response may buy you extra time, crucial time for your babies to develop and grow.

While contractions are the main indicator of preterm labor, you can't count on them to let you know what's going on. There are some other signs that indicate that labor is already in progress. Should you experience the following, notify your doctor immediately:

- Diarrhea
- Vaginal bleeding or discharge
- Uneasy sense that something is wrong

Some of these symptoms can be unrelated to preterm labor, but they should still be reported. Diarrhea and stomach upset can result from something you ate, but they can also be preliminaries to labor. Vaginal discharge is not an uncommon occurrence during pregnancy, but a change in the amount or type of discharge can be a warning sign. Any vaginal discharge that is bloody or streaked with blood can indicate that the cervix is beginning to dilate.

If you experience a leaking or gushing of fluid from the vagina, it could be a sign of premature rupture of membranes (PROM). The fluid comes from the amniotic sac that contains a baby. If that sac breaks open, the fluid will escape through your vagina. It might come out as a trickle or a gush, and it is usually clear with a distinct odor. A pH test can determine if it is indeed amniotic fluid, but you'll have to visit the doctor to confirm this. Even a small leak can present a danger of infection, so it's important to notify your caregiver as soon as possible.

PROM occurs in about ten percent of twin pregnancies, and more often in triplets or higher order multiples. Most multiples are in separate sacs, but some monozygotic twins are contained in a shared sac. One or all of the sacs may rupture prematurely, but it is usually the sac that is closest to the cervix.

Cerclage

If there is evidence that your cervix is shortening or dilating, an obstetrician may recommend a preventative procedure called a cerclage. Basically, cerclage involves sewing your cervix shut, keeping the babies inside until they're ready to be born. Sutures are inserted through the cervix to prevent it from opening; this can delay preterm birth and buy precious time for the babies to develop. It's more common with higher order multiples and in women whose previous pregnancy experience indicates an incompetent cervix.

Generally, cerclage is most effective when performed earlier in pregnancy. It may require a short period of hospitalization, during which contractions are monitored. You will be given anesthesia; generally, a spinal or epidural is used, but occasionally general anesthesia is warranted. After the procedure, you'll need to remain at the hospital for monitoring, perhaps for several hours or overnight. You may be given drugs to stave off infection or contractions. Once you return home, you should plan to take it easy for a couple of days, staying off your feet. There may be some mild bleeding, cramping, or vaginal discharge.

The cerclage sutures must be removed in order for you to deliver the babies vaginally. If the procedure is effective in staving off preterm labor, the sutures may be removed in the doctor's office at a time when it is determined that the babies are old enough for delivery—for example, thirty-six or thirty-seven weeks. Otherwise, they will be removed in the event of infection, when there are contractions indicating the immediate onset of labor, or if your water breaks.

Cerclage is not without risks. Most health professionals recognize that the benefits of prolonging pregnancy outweigh the risks, but you should still be aware of the potential consequences. They include:

- Preterm labor (the very thing you're trying to prevent)
- Chorioamnionitis, an infection of the amniotic sac
- Premature rupture of membranes (PROM)
- Laceration of the cervix
- Reaction to anesthesia or medication
- Hemorrhage

There is some disagreement as to whether cerclage actually has a positive impact. Some argue that if it extends pregnancy, even for a few weeks, then it benefits the babies. Others cite the associated risks and side effects and regard it as unnecessary intervention.

Your doctor may advise you to abstain from sexual intercourse before and after the cerclage due to the risk of introducing infection. Ask for specific advice as to when it is safe to resume sexual activity.

Treatment Options for Preterm Labor

If you are diagnosed with preterm labor, there are several options for treatment. Your doctor will first do an assessment of your condition. Your contractions will be monitored. Your cervix may be examined, and an ultrasound may be performed to update the status of the babies' development.

Ultimately, the goal of any treatment is to prevent or delay birth until the babies are developmentally ready. Treatment is an attempt to prolong pregnancy as long as possible, whether a matter of days, weeks, or months.

Rest and Relaxation

Often the first attempt to stop the progress of preterm labor is to assign the mother to rest. You may be encouraged to decrease your level of activity, or may need to begin some level of bed rest. Contractions will be monitored to see if they respond to the change in activity level. You may be given a monitor to use at home, or may be asked to report to the hospital or doctor's office for occasional monitoring. If dehydration is considered a factor, oral or intravenous fluid delivery may be required.

Treatment with Medication

There are a variety of drugs that can be used to counteract preterm labor and delay delivery. These medications, called tocolytics, act to relax the muscle of the uterus to stop it from contracting, or to counteract the hormones that are initiating the onset of labor.

There is some controversy regarding the use of tocolytic drugs. Currently, the FDA has not approved any drugs as effective in preventing preterm birth, but a category of drugs approved for other purposes may be prescribed. None of the choices are without side effects, however. You and your doctor will have to review the options and weigh the risks against the benefits.

Drugs such as terbutaline (also known as Brethine), ritodrine, nifedipine, and indomethacin are all used in treating preterm labor, although they were originally intended as medication for other conditions, such as asthma. While they are not approved by the FDA for use as tocolytics, they are the accepted standard of care in the medical field. Usually they are first administered intravenously, but are also available in the form of a pill or injection. Ongoing treatment may require the insertion of a subcutaneous pump to deliver small doses of the medicine at regular intervals. There is a great deal of controversy associated with the use of these pumps; be sure you fully discuss the risks and benefits of their use with your doctor, and consider alternatives.

ALERT!

All of these drugs have side effects and risks. Taking them is not generally a comfortable experience for the mother. Tocolytics can raise your heart rate, making you feel shaky and jittery. Headaches, dizziness, drowsiness, nausea, and muscle cramps may also result.

Magnesium sulfate is also commonly administered in the treatment of preterm labor. It's also used to treat preeclampsia and PIH (pregnancy-induced hypertension). It relaxes the muscles of the uterus. You will most likely be hospitalized for a few days while you receive this treatment so that you can be closely monitored for side effects. Magnesium sulfate can cause nausea, headache, weakness, and heart palpitations. Many women who take it experience a sensation of flushing and their skin feels hot.

Often, it is more effective to administer medication for the babies rather than the mother. Instead of slowing down labor, these drugs speed up the babies' development, increasing their viability at birth. In the last ten years, the use of corticosteroid therapy has greatly improved the odds for premature infants when administered twenty-four to forty-eight hours before birth. Steroids such as betamethasone or dexamethasone are injected into the mother to speed up the development of the babies' lungs and intestines to give them a better chance of survival after delivery.

Chapter 15

Labor with Multiples

After the long months of pregnancy, the onset of labor is the transition time marking the departure of pregnancy and the arrival of your babies. Whether your labor is long or short, weeks early or days overdue, it's an important process. It's the work your body must do to bring your babies to life.

Signs of Labor

Labor may come on suddenly, or it may take its time. Either way, you will want to know the signs so that you are ready to act at the appropriate time. Labor with twins, triplets, or more is not that much different than with a singleton; usually it starts out the same way, but requires more careful monitoring in case of complications. It also tends to happen earlier in pregnancy, so it may be unexpected. Being knowledgeable about the signs will give you confidence to act appropriately if you are surprised by early symptoms.

Contractions

The most important sign of labor is contractions. You may have been experiencing contractions earlier in your pregnancy, but labor contractions are different. You can distinguish them by their timing, regularity, and intensity. Productive contractions, those that are preparing your cervix for delivery, will come at regular intervals with increasing frequency. They will also increase in intensity.

ALERT!

Painless, irregular contractions that fade away if you lie down or change positions may be Braxton-Hicks, a form of "practice" contractions that ready your uterus for labor. With Braxton-Hicks, the sensation is usually centered in the abdomen, while true labor contractions may radiate from the front to the back.

Unless it is early in your pregnancy and your contractions are associated with preterm labor, or if you are in a great deal of discomfort or pain, you probably don't need to panic and rush to the hospital just yet. Use a stopwatch to gauge the amount of time in between the contraction sensations. Contact your doctor or midwife; they will advise you whether to head to the hospital or relax at home. They may suggest that you wait until your contractions reach a designated frequency, such as fifteen or twenty minutes apart, or recommend that you come in for monitoring. Because of the risk of complications, most health-care providers prefer to monitor multiple pregnancies more closely than singletons, and want expectant mothers of twins or more to arrive at the hospital earlier in the labor process.

Ruptured Membrane(s)

Another sign of labor is the release of fluid as the amniotic membrane ruptures or breaks. Despite the TV and movie stereotypes, you may not be fully aware if your water breaks. Rather than a gush and a splash, you might experience a trickle, and it can be difficult to ascertain whether it is labor or just a dribbling bladder.

However, if you have any suspicion that your water has broken, you should contact your doctor or midwife without delay. If the membranes have ruptured prematurely, you could be at risk for infection if delivery is not imminent. Usually, however, contractions follow shortly thereafter.

FACT

Many doctors recommend an induction of labor if contractions do not start within twenty-four or forty-eight hours after a woman's water breaks.

Other Signs

While regular, productive contractions are the sure sign of labor, there are several other symptoms that some women experience when it is almost time. They indicate that the body is getting ready for childbirth. Vaginal discharge that changes or increases could be a sign that your cervix is effacing or dilating, especially if it is accompanied by the bloody show, a plug of mucus from the cervix. It is sometimes accompanied by diarrhea. Discuss any of these symptoms with your medical caregiver if you suspect they are associated with the onset of labor.

At the Hospital: Examination and Preparation

When you arrive at the hospital, you will be examined to assess the progression of your labor. If it's determined that your contractions are "false labor" because your cervix is not opening, you may be sent home, a disappointing and frustrating experience after the excitement of arriving at the hospital. However, in a multiple pregnancy, many doctors prefer to keep a closer eye on their patients, and may recommend you remain at the hospital for monitoring.

Many hospitals allow mothers of multiples to labor in a labor suite, outfitted with more comfortable amenities than a standard hospital room. However, don't get too comfortable. It is common to move mothers of multiples to an operating room before delivery, in case there is a need for emergency cesarean surgery. Check with the facility where you will deliver about their policies so you know what to expect.

You will probably have an IV or heparin lock inserted in the event that medication or a hydrating solution is required. You'll change into a gown, either one you've brought from home or one provided by the hospital. Finally, you and the babies will be monitored. With one monitor per baby, and one for your contractions, you may feel a bit overwired. Be sure to read the information on monitoring later in this chapter, so that you understand all of your options.

Inducing Labor

There are some instances where labor doesn't start on its own and it needs to be artificially initiated. There are many reasons why medical professionals may recommend inducing labor, but ultimately the decision is made because the babies or their mother will be better off if the babies are born rather than remaining in the womb. Sometimes it is because one or both babies are in distress, perhaps due to cord compression, placenta malfunction, or infection. In other situations, the mother's well-being is at risk, such as when preeclampsia develops.

E
ALERT!

Your doctor may recommend induction at thirty-seven or thirty-eight weeks if you have not delivered your twins prior to that date, or she may prefer to wait until forty weeks to provide additional time for you to start labor on your own.

Ways to Induce Labor

There are a couple of different ways to prompt labor, and the approach will depend on the reasons motivating the induction and on your physical condition. Induction serves to ripen the cervix and stimulate contractions. This can be achieved manually or by administering hormones.

Often, the first step is to apply prostaglandin, which contains a hormone associated with labor, to the cervix. It is applied in a fairly quick and painless procedure, and has the effect of softening the cervical tissue so that it can better respond to the contractions. Prostaglandin may be applied the day before a scheduled induction as the first in a series of treatments. Or it may be sufficient to prompt the onset of labor on its own.

In cases where the amniotic sac(s) remain intact, another way to induce labor is to manually strip the membranes by loosening the bag of waters from the wall of the uterus. Doing so may help start labor by releasing prostaglandins and allowing the first baby to rest directly on the cervix, pressuring it to expand and open. However, it also presents a risk of infection, and doesn't provide any guarantees that labor will result.

Labor can also be induced by administering Pitocin, a synthetic form of the pregnancy hormone oxytocin, to start or strengthen contractions. Pitocin is delivered intravenously, and may require incremental increases to produce effective contractions. For some women, labor induced by Pitocin may result in intensified contractions. You'll be monitored closely to ensure that the contractions don't stress the babies.

There are also some natural methods of prompting labor. You should discuss these options with your medical caregiver before attempting them, but they may be worth considering before attempting a medical induction. Stimulating your nipples or having sexual intercourse to the point of orgasm may sufficiently raise your own hormones and prompt contractions.

A less pleasant tradition is to swallow castor oil, a potent laxative, to activate your bowels.

Impact of Induction

Induction is not always a direct route to delivery. Induced labor may be longer or more intense than spontaneous labor, or it may fail altogether. Induction is associated with a higher rate of cesarean delivery. Your doctor may recommend a cesarean if your labor doesn't adequately progress after a designated trial, perhaps twenty-four hours.

FACT

Induction of labor is on the rise in the United States. The Centers for Disease Control and Prevention reported that more than 20 percent of babies were delivered after induction in 2002. That's nearly double the rate reported in 1989, when only 9 percent of women were induced before delivery.

Stages of Labor

The process of childbirth can be broken down into three stages. The first stage, the process of opening the cervix, is generally the longest and most uncomfortable stage. The good news about labor with multiples is that the hard work accomplished by the body during this stage accommodates both (or all) babies; you don't have to repeat this stage for each baby. Understanding the process, and knowing what to expect, can help you manage your expectations and create a more meaningful experience.

During the first stage, the cervix must fully open as a passageway for the babies. This stage can be broken down into three phases, which are covered in detail here. The final stages of childbirth, pushing and delivery of the placenta, will be discussed in the next chapter.

First Phase: Early (Latent) Labor

Early, or latent, labor is the first phase of the first stage of labor. It is during this time that the cervix prepares to open and provide access for the babies' departure from the womb. This readying of the cervix is called ripening, and it requires the cervix to do two things: efface (thin out) and dilate (open).

You can be in early labor for several days, or even weeks, without really being aware of it. Gentle contractions and pressure on the cervix open it a couple of centimeters. They may be as infrequent as once an hour, but will occur with increasing frequency and will intensify as the phase progresses. They can last as long as forty-five seconds each. Most women are fairly comfortable through this stage, and are able to participate in light activity.

Latent labor lasts, on average, for ten to twelve hours. For women experiencing childbirth for the first time, it can be longer. However, the extra weight and pressure associated with carrying two or more babies often expedites the process for mothers of multiples.

Second Phase: Active Labor

Early labor gives way to the active phase when the contractions are about five minutes apart and the cervix has dilated to three or four centimeters. The contractions are intense at this point, lasting up to a full minute, but with breaks in between. A mother in this phase of labor will become increasingly uncomfortable, and will need assistance to manage the pain, either with medication or relaxation techniques.

While it may have taken twelve hours for the cervix to dilate a couple of centimeters during the latent phase, the increased contractions and pressure of the baby moving toward the birth canal speed up the process during active labor. It can take only a few hours or as little as fifteen minutes for the cervix to fully dilate to ten centimeters. If labor stalls during this phase, Pitocin may be administered to jump-start the process.

A doula or labor coach begins to play a very supportive role during this portion of labor, helping the mother to focus her energy during the contractions and keeping her comfortable and relaxed during breaks.

Phase Three: Transition

Just when you think that you can't take any more, the final phase of labor intensifies your discomfort. Contractions lasting more than a minute come fast and furious, as frequently as every other minute. The presenting baby's proximity to your fully dilated cervix places increasing pressure on your bottom. You may feel like you want to push, but will have to focus your energy on resisting the urge, according to your doctor's or midwife's direction. To make matters worse, your body may betray you, compounding your discomfort with nausea, vomiting, and pressure in your rectum.

In the midst of this discomfort, you will likely be moved to an operating room or a delivery room equipped for emergency surgery. That's a good sign; it means that the arrival of your babies is not far away!

Monitoring

With more than one baby in the mix, the risk of complications for one or all of them is heightened. To control the risk, the medical community is generally more comfortable with close monitoring of babies during the labor process. Therefore, you are more likely than a mother of a singleton to be monitored during your labor. You should be aware of your options for monitoring, discuss them with your doctor, and include references to your wishes in your birth plan.

Fetal monitoring is used to record the patterns of each baby's heartbeat to detect changes in the rhythm or frequency that might indicate distress. A normal fetal heart beats between 120 and 160 times per minute.

Fetal Monitoring

There are two ways to keep an eye on the babies' condition while they're still in the womb; external and internal fetal monitoring.

If your babies will be externally monitored, electronic sensors will be attached to your belly with straps. Some models may have two or more sensors for multiples, or multiple units will be put in place. The sensors will be positioned directly over each fetus to monitor the beat of each heart. The monitors are connected to a machine that prints out a graph. The output doesn't look like much more than an ongoing jagged line, but your healthcare provider will be able to see if the babies' heart rates are above or below the norm, indicating a lack of oxygen or other signs of distress.

As the babies wiggle around in your womb, they may move out of the range of their sensors, causing the signal to be lost. This isn't a sign of distress, but it may be necessary to reposition the sensors. Sometimes the monitor is connected to an alarm that sounds when the reading exceeds acceptable levels. This alarm can be somewhat of an annoying disturbance, especially when it is triggered by a false reading.

Internal monitoring is more precise, and avoids the false alarms of disrupted external readings. A small electrode will be inserted into your womb through an opening in the cervix and attached to a baby's scalp. This can only be accomplished if the head is accessible, so the bag of waters will be broken if it is still intact. It requires the mother to be immobile for the remainder of labor, so it's usually reserved when there is great cause for concern. Also, it's difficult to monitor multiples with an internal monitor, as it only accesses the presenting baby—that is, the one closest to the cervix. So external monitoring is a more likely option.

Monitoring Contractions

In addition to keeping a close eye on the babies, your contractions will be monitored. This may seem redundant to you; after all, you will probably be painfully aware of each contraction as it happens. But it is still important to assess the frequency and intensity of the contractions in order to determine how well labor is progressing. Even if pain medication dulls your perception, the monitor will help your caregivers keep track of the exact frequency and duration of each contraction. It can be particularly important if you are induced, to ensure that the right dosage of Pitocin is administered.

Contractions are monitored using a sensor that senses the changes in the surface of your abdomen. It will generate a graph printout similar to the fetal heart rate. Like a fetal monitor, this monitor's signal can be disrupted by movement. A more accurate assessment can be obtained with an intrauterine-pressure catheter (IUPC) to measure the actual pressure within the uterus.

Wireless monitors provide continuous assessment without inhibiting movement. Called telemetry, this advanced technology combines the best of both worlds, giving mothers more control over their body during labor, but allowing doctors to keep a close eye on the babies.

Monitoring Alternatives

Continuous monitoring can be uncomfortable and inconvenient for a mother in labor. With her movement restricted by belts, straps, and wires, she's prevented from physically working through her contractions. If your pregnancy and labor have proceeded without complications, you may be able to consider some alternatives that would allow you more freedom to labor comfortably. Your doula can act as an advocate if you wish to pursue another option.

One alternative to continuous monitoring is intermittent assessments of the babies' heart rates. A nurse or midwife can take a reading of the babies' conditions using a stethoscope or handheld ultrasound at designated intervals—for example, every fifteen minutes. With this method, it is important to ensure that each individual baby's heartbeat is able to be detected and receives equal attention.

Pain Management During Labor

There's no way around it, the process of labor can be quite painful. While labor with multiples is not necessarily more painful than with a singleton, there are some special concerns regarding the ways that pain is managed.

Medical Pain Management

Medications to dull or block sensations of pain may make the labor experience much more comfortable. While there are some risks associated with anesthesia, modern options for pain relief are generally very safe for both the mother and the babies.

Many women sing the praises of epidurals for the relief that they can provide during childbirth. In the event that a c-section is warranted, the epidural can also be used to administer anesthesia for the surgery. The only downside to epidural pain management is in the installation; once in place, an epidural delivers immediate, continuous pain relief to the lower half of your body without impacting your mental acuity.

A small percentage of mothers suffer from headaches after an epidural. You can reduce the risk of this side effect by remaining perfectly still during the insertion.

Inserting an epidural requires the presence of an anesthesiologist, as well as your cooperation to sit perfectly still with your back exposed to provide access to your spine. After an injection with a numbing solution, the anesthesiologist will insert a catheter into the hollow space just outside the membrane surrounding your spine at your lower back. The procedure takes about fifteen minutes.

With the catheter in place, pain relief can be administered, usually a combination of narcotics and local anesthetics. Although the cocktail blocks the sensation of pain, you'll retain control of your lower body. It may make you unsteady on your feet, however.

For a rapid, short burst of pain relief, a spinal block can deliver immediate results. It works much like an epidural, but the anesthesia is injected directly into the spinal fluid rather than through a catheter. It's quicker to administer than an epidural, but only provides a limited one-shot dose of relief, so it's only used in circumstances where the mother isn't likely to require pain medication for an extended amount of time. Another option is a combination epidural/spinal block. It requires one insertion, but gives you the option of either immediate or extended delivery of anesthesia.

Early in labor, systemic medications, such as Stadol or Demerol, can help take the edge off the pain. They'll be administered through your IV or injected. They won't make the pain disappear, but can dull the sensation enough to help you relax. These drugs will probably make you drowsy, and the babies as well, since they can enter the fetal circulation through the placenta. For that reason, the effects are short-lived, and they should only be given in early labor, long before delivery is imminent.

FACT

If you attended a childbirth education class, you likely learned several nonmedical strategies for managing the pain and discomfort of labor. A doula or labor partner may be able to assist you in implementing them. Breath control, relaxation, massage, and other means of providing comfort can help reduce or delay your need for medical pain relief.

Unmedicated "Natural" Birth

A multiple birth free of medical intervention is fairly rare. Despite a trend toward "natural," unmedicated childbirth, few mothers of multiples deliver their babies without anesthesia. Many of those who do, do so unintentionally, either because their labor progresses too quickly or some other complications prevent the opportunity to administer it. If it is your goal to deliver without pain medication, discuss your wishes with your doctor. Hiring a doula to assist you through the experience may be a worthwhile investment.

You may wish to consider having a catheter implanted just in case, so that regional anesthesia can be administered in the event of an emergency c-section or if the pain becomes unbearable. Otherwise, you may miss the birth entirely due to being unconscious from general anesthesia.

Chapter 16

Delivering Your Babies

The time has come! Your babies are making their entry into this world. Whether you deliver vaginally or via cesarean section, delivering twins, triplets, or higher order multiples is an amazing event, leading up to the miraculous moment when you meet your babies face-to-face for the first time.

Presentation Combinations

An important factor in delivering multiples is presentation, the term used to describe the position of the babies within the womb. The presentation of the babies at the time of delivery will guide your doctors in deciding the best method of delivery. There are several combinations of positions that your babies can take.

Vertex / Vertex

Vertex / Breech

◀ The babies may be in a variety of positions, or presentations.

Breech / Vertex

Breech / Breech

Vertex / Transverse

Breech / Transverse

Vertex is the term to describe a baby that is resting head-down, the most common and safest option for vaginal delivery. Your doctor will be most concerned with whether the presenting baby—that is, the one closest to the cervix—is vertex, as this is the baby that would enter the birth canal first. A twin pregnancy where both babies are vertex is the best candidate for a vaginal birth.

A breech baby is the opposite of a vertex baby; his head is pointing upright. A breech baby may be arranged in one of three ways:

- **Frank breech:** The buttocks are positioned closest to the cervix, with the legs folded straight up toward the head.
- **Complete breech:** The buttocks are pointed toward the cervix, but the arms and legs are crossed in front of the body.
- **Incomplete or footling breech:** One or both legs are dangling down toward the cervix.

There is some controversy as to the best option for delivering a breech baby. Some doctors are more comfortable performing a cesarean section if even one of the babies is breech. Others are willing to attempt a breech delivery if certain conditions are met.

Transverse babies rest horizontally in the womb. A transverse baby lying at the bottom of the womb is not a good candidate for a vaginal delivery. Usually, however, the baby closest to the cervix is either breech or vertex and the second baby rests in a transverse position higher in the womb, close to the mother's rib cage. Your doctor will most likely base a delivery decision on the position of the presenting baby.

Is Vaginal Delivery an Option for You?

Delivery through the birth canal and out the vagina is generally the safest method of birth for mother and babies, and therefore it is the preferred approach, unless certain circumstances create risks that make a cesarean section a better option. Vaginal delivery carries less risk of hemorrhage or infection, requires less anesthesia, and has a quicker recovery time. It also produces less scarring.

The babies may also benefit from a vaginal delivery. As they travel through the birth canal, their lungs are compressed, forcing out fluid and preparing them to breathe air.

Vaginal delivery is not an option if

- You are having triplets, quadruplets, or other higher order multiples.
- Your twins are monoamniotic (share an amniotic sac).
- The presentation of either baby is transverse lie.
- You have active genital herpes.
- Your have placenta previa or another medical condition.
- Your pelvic structure makes it difficult for your babies to pass through.

Vaginal delivery may be discouraged if

- One or both babies is breech.
- You have preeclampsia.
- One or more of the babies are in severe distress and cannot tolerate labor.
- Previous cesarean delivery or abdominal surgery puts you at risk for uterine rupture.

Vaginal Birth after Cesarean (VBAC)

At one time, a previous cesarean section automatically ruled out a vaginal delivery. That is not the case these days, however. The danger of labor and delivery after cesarean surgery is that the incision site could rupture. New techniques make that less likely now. Most doctors are willing to attempt a VBAC (short for vaginal birth after cesarean), as long as certain conditions are met.

It's important for your doctor or midwife to review your case if you have had a previous c-section, so be sure they are aware of your history. While in most cases a VBAC is feasible, the extra strain that multiples place on your uterus may make it too risky.

Breech Babies

Breech babies are the source of some contention among the medical community. Only a small percentage of singleton babies are presenting breech at delivery and, in most cases, a decision is made to schedule a cesarean section to deliver those babies. However, opinions differ on the appropriate approach for breech twins. Believing that most multiples are smaller than singletons of the same gestational age, some doctors are actually more willing to deliver a breech twin than a singleton. It is only rarely favorable to deliver vaginally if the presenting baby is breech. However, a breech baby following a vertex twin may be a candidate for vaginal delivery.

Sometimes the doctor or midwife will make an attempt to turn the breech baby. If unsuccessful, consideration will be given to the baby's status. Is he tolerating the labor well? Does he appear to be in any distress? Is he frank breech, the least difficult position to deliver? Fetal monitoring and ultrasound will give a picture of the baby's condition.

ALERT!

Even identical twins can look very different at birth when one is vertex and the other is delivered breech. A vertex baby's head is rounded by its headfirst passage through the birth canal, while a breech baby's head is more pointy and cone-shaped. After birth, the soft skull tissue reforms into a normal shape and they will look more alike.

One of the most important criteria to consider in determining whether a baby should be delivered breech is how her size compares to her co-twin. If the second baby is smaller than the first, she is more likely to be a successful breech delivery, as the doctor can be fairly assured that she will pass through the birth canal.

Your doctor's previous experience will determine his comfort level with breech delivery. If your baby meets the criteria to attempt a breech delivery, your doctor will reach into your womb and grab the baby's feet, you'll push and he'll pull, and the baby will slip feet-first through your cervix and into the world.

Vaginal Delivery: Pushing

The process of labor, described in the previous chapter, prepares the mother's body for a vaginal delivery. After the first stage of labor completely opens the cervix to provide a gateway for the baby's exit from the womb, it's time for the second stage of labor: pushing the presenting baby through the pelvic bones and out the vaginal opening. This stage can last for five minutes or several hours. Usually, it lasts about an hour. On average, it takes three to five pushes to move the baby out.

After the fast and frequent contractions experienced during the transition part of the first stage, this second stage of labor provides some relative relief. However, while the contractions may subside somewhat in frequency, they won't lessen in intensity, and they will be accompanied by an overwhelming urge to push or bear down. Your doctor or midwife may guide you to coordinate your pushing efforts with your contractions, or you may be encouraged to bear down when it feels right. If your epidural is still effective, you should probably receive some coaching, as your sensation will be dulled.

The force of your uterus's contractions will continue to force the baby through your pelvis toward the vaginal opening. If necessary, an episiotomy will be performed to prevent tearing of the perineum. The doctor will make a small cut to the tissue that stretches between your vagina and rectum. The clean cut heals faster than ripped tissue. Or perineal massage may help stretch the tissue to accommodate the oncoming baby.

The bad news: You have to experience this stage of labor separately with each baby. The good news: Twins are usually a bit smaller than singleton babies and most mothers of multiples don't have a difficult time pushing them out.

Once the head crowns, or bulges through the perineum, the excitement really begins. Your doctor or midwife will slowly coach the first baby's head out of your vagina. You may be instructed to stop pushing for a moment while her nose and mouth are suctioned. After the head, the largest part of the baby's body, has exited, the arms, torso, and legs slip out without much exertion. The umbilical cord will be clamped and cut, and your first twin will be handed off to a waiting attendant.

It's done! The first baby has arrived! You can bask in the joy of this moment and relax for a few moments. You're not completely finished yet, though. There's more to come.

The Intermission: Between Babies

If you were having a singleton, your childbirth experience would end here. But you're having another baby! While twins may be born within a few minutes of each other, most twins arrive at intervals of twenty to thirty minutes. This intermission between babies is a crucial time, during which both babies' condition will be assessed.

With more room to move, the second baby may stretch out and change position—with luck, into a vertex presentation. His rearrangement will likely be monitored by ultrasound to determine the course of action. If the baby is in a breech or transverse position, your doctor may attempt to turn him. This process, called external cephalic version, can be uncomfortable, as the doctor pushes forcefully on your abdomen in an attempt to turn the baby head down.

FACT

There have been some cases where twins or other multiples experience an extended intermission between births. Usually this occurs when preterm labor cannot be halted and one multiple is delivered extremely prematurely. In a delayed interval birth, the labor is stopped after the birth of one fetus, and a cerclage is performed to close the cervix. This gives the remaining baby or babies more time to develop and optimizes their chances for survival.

This baby requires some careful monitoring during this time. If his bag of water remained intact during the delivery of his co-twin, it will need to be broken now. With his brother or sister out of the way, his situation poses some risk. The previous contractions and pushing activity may have caused the placenta to detach, reducing the amount of oxygen delivered to the remaining baby. And there is always a concern about cord compression or prolapse, if the umbilical cord enters the birth canal before the baby does.

Your contractions will also be watched carefully during this time. If your uterus slacks off, you may receive a dose of Pitocin to reactivate the contractions to deliver the second baby. If everything is in place, it's time to push out the second baby. With a path already paved by her co-twin, the good news is that the second twin usually requires fewer pushes and is often born relatively quickly.

Final Stage: Delivery of the Placenta(s)

After both babies are delivered, there's one final step. You have to deliver the placenta(s). This important organ has been the source of nutrition and nourishment for your babies for the last few months, but now that it is no longer needed, it is time for it to depart your womb.

Your contractions will continue, with a different purpose. Instead of dilating your cervix or forcing out a baby, these contractions serve to separate the placenta from the uterine wall. A final push will expel it through your vagina. Fused or single placentas will be delivered in one shot. If your babies had separate placentas, you may have to go through this process more than once.

ESSENTIAL

Most hospitals do so as a matter of routine, but you'll want the placenta(s) sent to pathology for examination. An analysis may reveal your babies' zygosity. A monochorionic placenta will indicate that your twins are monozygotic, or identical.

When the doctor or midwife clamps each cord, request that they distinguish the cords—and the corresponding placentas—so that they can be identified for ownership. In the event that there is a problem with one of the babies, an examination of cord or placental abnormalities might help pinpoint a diagnosis.

With your hard work done, you can lie back and relax. If you were given an episiotomy or experienced any tearing, you'll be stitched up and cleaned up. Your epidural may be removed at this time if you don't require any follow-up care.

Cesarean Section

Nearly all triplets, quadruplets, and higher order multiples are delivered by cesarean section. About 50 percent of twin pregnancies are candidates for cesarean delivery. Your cesarean delivery may not be a surprise. With multiples, it is often a planned event, decided in advance based on your situation. Even if you prefer a vaginal delivery, you should consider the possibility of a c-section and prepare accordingly.

Why Cesarean?

A cesarean section may be planned due to anticipated complications for you or your babies. This is the case when there are higher order multiples, monoamniotic twins, placenta previa, or other conditions that would make a vaginal delivery dangerous. Other times, your doctor may decide that a c-section is the best course of action after labor has started, perhaps because of the babies' presentation or because monitoring indicates that they are not tolerating the pressure of the uterine contractions. Finally, sometimes an emergency cesarean must be performed despite the mother's best efforts to deliver vaginally, because of fetal distress or other dire consequences that could result in the loss of mother or babies if delivery is not immediate.

Preparing for a Cesarean

If your c-section is planned, once being admitted to the hospital you will be prepped for surgery in the operating room. In most cases, you can be accompanied by your husband, partner, or birth coach. Certified doulas are usually allowed to attend as well, but hospital policies vary on this issue. An intravenous line will be established and the area of your abdomen sterilized and possibly shaved. A catheter will be inserted to keep your bladder empty.

Except in the case of emergency c-sections, you will be given regional anesthesia, which will allow you to be awake and alert during the procedure without feeling any sensation in the lower half of your body. Anesthesia is generally administered with a spinal or epidural. A nasal cannula fitted in your nostrils will provide oxygen for you to breathe. The babies will be monitored with ultrasound and fetal monitoring, and your vital signs will be continuously checked.

A sterile environment is imperative in the operating room. Your body will be draped with sterile cloths. A screen will prevent you from viewing the actual procedure, but may be lowered to show you the babies as they are removed from the womb. Your husband or partner will also have to don a surgical scrub suit, mask, and hair and shoe coverings to accompany you in the operating room.

E ALERT!

Hospital policies vary regarding the use of cameras in the operating room. Be sure you investigate the rules beforehand to find out which aspects of the birth can be filmed. By all means, check your camera's supply of batteries, film, or memory storage ahead of time. You don't want to miss the big moment because of an equipment malfunction!

Emotionally, you may feel anxious, excited, terrified, and elated. Physically, while you won't feel the pain of the procedure, you may feel somewhat uncomfortable lying flat on your back. You may feel vulnerable and intimidated by the strange sights and busy activity surrounding you. You may feel nauseous from the effects of the anesthesia or your prone position, and may even have to retch or vomit. Your anesthesiologist may be able to help you overcome this feeling with medication added to your IV.

The Section

Fortunately, the procedure itself is relatively short. The doctor will make an incision low across the pubic area; this "bikini cut" creates a less conspicuous scar and reduces the risk of uterine complications in future pregnancies. After cutting through muscle and tissue to access the uterus, the doctor will make an incision through the uterine wall to access the first baby. As the baby is lifted out, you may feel some pressure and tugging, but no pain.

As the baby is lifted out, ask to have the screen lowered so that you can have a look. The baby's cord will be clamped and cut, and the baby will be handed to an attendant for examination. In the meantime, the doctor will already be moving on to the next baby, reaching into your uterus and pulling out another multiple. Another attendant will be ready to receive her, and the process will continue until all the babies have been delivered. You may be able to hear your babies cry out as they take their first breaths. Your partner may have the opportunity to participate in the process, cutting the cords or holding the babies after they have been examined.

After the babies are removed from your womb, your doctor will deliver the placenta(s) and examine your uterus for fragments of placental tissue. A dose of Pitocin in your IV will help your overworked uterus start the road to recovery. Then the process of suturing and stitching begins, which often takes longer than the actual delivery.

FACT

During pregnancy, babies are often identified as "Baby A," "Baby B," "Baby C," and so forth based on their presentation, with the baby closest to the cervix termed Baby A. In a cesarean delivery, the babies may or may not arrive in order, depending on how they are arranged in the womb. The baby closest to the incision will be the first to be born.

Emergency C-Section/Combination Birth

Many mothers are very concerned about the prospect of delivering their first baby vaginally and then having a c-section to deliver the second baby, as it means experiencing the worst sensations of both methods: suffering through the discomfort of labor as well as surgery, and having to recover from both an episiotomy and an incision. While you'll probably hear plenty of stories about this unfortunate series of events in twin birth, statistically it's not likely to happen. Only 15 percent of twin births happen in this fashion.

No doctor prefers this combined method of delivery. If there is any doubt that the second baby can be delivered vaginally, a cesarean section would be recommended to begin with. Surgery to deliver the second baby is only performed when fetal distress is indicated and the baby's life is at risk. Although it is not the ideal experience, most mothers would agree that their baby's life is worth the added discomfort.

The Babies' First Few Moments

No matter how you deliver, your babies will spend their first few moments amid a whirlwind of activity. Most deliveries of twins or more will be attended by an array of medical staff. Often the babies are well outnumbered by their attendants, with at least one doctor and nurse caring for each infant.

Immediately after birth, your babies' condition will be assessed. After placing them on a warming tray and cleaning them up, the medical staff will be checking out several different aspects of their physical state. Your babies' first standardized test is the Apgar, which provides a general assessment of their health at birth. Apgar is assessed twice, when they are one minute old and then again, five minutes later.

A score of ten is perfect, and anything above seven is considered average. If there is cause for concern based on a lower score, your baby will be treated according to his needs.

Infant Apgar Assessment

Characteristic	What It Measures	0	1	2
Activity Level	Muscle Tone	Limp	Some	Active
Pulse	Heart Rate	Absent	Slow	Above 100 bpm
Grimace	Reflex Irritability	None	Grimace	Cough or sneeze
Appearance	Skin Color	Blue or pale	Body pink, extremities blue	Pink
Respiration	Breathing	Absent	Weak	Good

In addition, your babies will be weighed and measured. Ointment or eyedrops will be placed in their eyes. Their footprints will be inked, and a blood sample will be taken for testing. They'll be given a dose of vitamin K to assist with blood clotting. Depending on their condition, as well as your recovery status, the babies may spend some time in your arms. This quiet period of alertness that follows birth is an ideal time to initiate breastfeeding.

If your babies are born early, the events of their birth may be surrounded by a bit more concern and immediacy. Neonatologists will be standing by to care for them as they make their entry. Quick action will be taken to ease their transition from the womb to the world, especially to help them breathe. They may be whisked away to the NICU (neonatal intensive care unit), and your opportunity to spend time with them may be limited as the medical staff strives to stabilize them.

The abrupt end to your pregnancy can be a very difficult experience. Your babies may be facing several months of critical care. However, many premature infants survive their ominous start in life; only time will tell your babies' stories. Have faith in the medical staff's ability to care for them. You'll find much more information on parenting premature multiples in Chapter 17.

Postpartum Care and Recovery

Just as your body—and mind—took some time to adjust to the idea of being pregnant, you'll need some time to recover after giving birth. Your recovery period will be determined by how you delivered; cesarean moms have undergone major surgery and will need more time to heal, although a vaginal delivery also takes a toll on a woman's body.

After Vaginal Delivery

After delivery, your uterus will begin to shrink back to its pre-pregnancy size. You may feel some mild cramping during this process, but you should not experience extreme discomfort. If you do, notify your doctor. You'll have some bleeding, which may be heavy at first. For the first few days you may find that you soak a sanitary napkin in a couple of hours. If you've had a previous pregnancy, you won't find this surprising, but it may be heavier than you experienced in the past. That's because your uterus stretched and expanded further to accommodate the extra babies. You may want to be prepared with some supersize sanitary napkins from home; they'll work better than those provided by the hospital.

ALERT!

Drinking plenty of fluids is vital after delivery, especially if you intend to nurse your babies. An increased fluid intake will speed your recovery and keep you healthy as you begin to care for your newborns.

The bloody discharge, called lochia, can last for several weeks after delivery. It should taper off, however, and should not include any large clumps or clots. If it increases, or is accompanied by pain, fever, or a foul odor, notify your doctor right away.

You will need to wear sanitary napkins to accommodate this discharge for up to six weeks after you deliver. Tampons are not recommended. If you experienced anemia during your pregnancy, it's important to continue supplementing your iron intake, either by eating iron-rich foods or by taking pills prescribed by your doctor.

If you had an episiotomy or any tearing of the perineum during your delivery, you may be somewhat sore. Ice packs, sitz baths, and witch-hazel pads can relieve the discomfort. You may also be plagued by hemorrhoids as your distended veins return to normal capacity. Discuss their treatment with your caregiver.

Although you'll probably be ready to leave the hospital soon after your delivery, it will take a couple of weeks for your body to return to full strength. After the strain of pregnancy, the process of labor is intense—your body worked hard!—and you need to give yourself time to recuperate. It's not realistic to expect that you will get plenty of rest and relaxation; the weeks following the delivery of multiples are hectic, to say the least. But you should definitely consider lining up plenty of help so that you can minimize your responsibilities and focus your energy exclusively on caring for yourself and the babies.

After C-Section

A cesarean section is major surgery, and necessitates more intensive recovery. You'll probably have to remain in bed for at least twelve hours, after which time you'll be encouraged to move around or at least get out of bed. It may be unpleasant; the effects of the surgery and the anesthesia may leave you feeling like you've been hit by a truck. Rely on the nurses and caregivers to assist you. You may have a great deal of pain or discomfort, but relief is available. Discuss your options for pain medication with your doctor.

QUESTION?

Will pain medications affect my breastfeeding plans?
You can still initiate breastfeeding, even if you are taking pain medication. You doctor will advise you if the medication will impact the babies. Even if it prevents you from feeding the babies, you can still begin the nursing process using a pump.

A cesarean section does not exempt you from the other aftereffects of delivering a baby. You will still have some cramping as your uterus returns to its normal size, and you will have a vaginal discharge of lochia as your body expels blood and tissue. As with a vaginal delivery, you'll have to wear sanitary napkins for several weeks after your babies are born.

As you recover from a c-section, you'll have to avoid strenuous activity for a period of time. That may include driving, stair climbing, and heavy lifting. Depending on your circumstances, it may be difficult to obey some of these restrictions. However, it is important to follow your doctor's recommendations during your recovery. You cannot effectively care for your newborns if you are unwell. Arrange for extra help and give your body the time and nurturing it needs to heal.

Emotional Impact

No matter how much you read, study, and prepare for the arrival of your babies, their birth will be nothing like you expected. You may feel overwhelmed by emotions: relief, anxiety, elation, despair, fear, and love. Your conflicting feelings may stir up some unusual reactions. Remember that this is a time of transition. You're not pregnant with multiples any more; rather, you are the mother of two, three, or more infants. You are all settling into your new roles as a family and will require some time to adjust.

Postpartum depression (PPD) is characterized by feelings of hopelessness that last most of the day, and don't diminish after several weeks. It's normal to feel overwhelmed or out of control, but you need to seek medical attention if your feelings are preventing you from properly caring for your babies or yourself.

Fifteen percent of women experience postpartum depression after giving birth, and mothers of twins or more are particularly at risk. A 2004 study by the National Organization of Mothers of Twins Clubs found that nearly 40 percent of moms of multiples experienced depression.

Have some strategies in place for coping with the stress of multiples. Line up plenty of help to see you through the rough times. Maintain a sense of humor. Find the joy in your amazing babies. Establish priorities and give yourself permission to temporarily release any nonessential responsibilities.

Communication is key. Talk to your spouse or partner about your feelings. Share your experience with fellow parents of multiples; they will understand what you're going through. Down the road, you will recall the rush of emotion that followed the birth of your babies with amazing tenderness.

Chapter 17

Premature Multiples

Prematurity is a reality for many multiples. While it's not the ideal way to begin life, these babies are remarkably adaptive and can usually overcome their early start after a few weeks in the hospital. Premature babies will require specialized medical care. It's not the most pleasant experience for babies, or their parents, and it's a difficult topic to talk about. Nevertheless, it's vitally important for parents of multiples to understand the ramifications of prematurity in the event that their babies do arrive early.

The Impact of Premature Birth

Normally, human babies require about 270 days to fully develop in the womb, after which they are usually ready to make the transition to life on the outside. When babies are born too early, many of their body's organs and systems are immature, unable to function properly on their own. Fortunately, medical science has the ability to help those babies stay alive until they can sustain themselves.

The consequences of premature birth vary from short-term to long-lasting. Some are major disabilities while others are minor inconveniences. Some are manifested immediately while others may not surface until later in life. How prematurity will affect your babies depends a great deal on just how early they were born. For example, cerebral palsy, mental retardation, and blindness are all major complications that result from premature birth. At the other end of the spectrum are minor conditions that can be corrected or overcome later in life, such as asthma, vision deficiencies, hyperactivity, or orthopedic irregularities.

Preemie Viability

Weeks Gestation	Survival Rate	Impact
23 weeks	30% survive	100% of survivors have major disability
24 weeks	60–65% survive	40–50% have major disability
25 weeks	70% survive	Varies depending on complications
26 weeks	75% survive	Varies depending on complications
28 weeks and up	80%+ survive	Varies depending on complications
29–34 weeks	90% survive	Minimal

Birth is the transition point between development in the womb and life on the outside. Premature babies simply aren't ready to exist in the outside world. Fortunately, medical intervention makes it possible to sustain their vital systems while the babies adapt to the conditions of life and finish developing outside the womb. However, their immature functioning can often cause irreparable damage to vital organs.

One of the most difficult aspects of having premature babies is not knowing where they will land within the spectrum of severity. There is simply no way to know what the future holds. Only time will reveal the full impact of prematurity on your multiples.

FACT

About twenty years ago, babies born prior to twenty-eight weeks gestation were not considered viable. However, advances in medical technology now make it possible for some infants as young as twenty-three weeks to survive. For each week that the baby is denied development in the womb, the chances of catastrophic complications increase.

Medical Issues of Premature Birth

Preemie babies face such a daunting array of challenges. Nearly every physical system is affected. Some of the issues can be addressed medically, with drugs, treatments, and even surgery. Others simply require the passage of time and will resolve with maturation.

Respiratory Problems

Breathing is the biggest problem for premature infants. Without breath, the intake of oxygen and outflow of carbon dioxide, a human simply can't live. Designed to function in the fluid-filled environment of the womb, preemie babies' lungs just can't make the immediate transition to air; they're almost like a fish out of water.

Helping your babies breathe is a critical step in stabilizing them after birth. Initially, a hand bag can be used for artificial respiration until the babies are intubated, or placed on a ventilator. The ventilator, also called a respirator, essentially does the breathing for them, forcing air in and out of their lungs. Some babies will need to breathe air with a higher concentration of oxygen until their lungs mature enough to tolerate the air around them. The ventilator may mimic the physical process of breathing for your babies, but eventually their brain must take over the operation, reminding them to breathe on their own.

One of the major causes of respiratory distress in premature infants is the lack of surfactant, a component in the lungs that makes breathing easier. Just as stretching out a balloon makes it easier to blow up, surfactant makes the lungs more elastic and easier to fill with air. Administration of synthetic surfactant greatly enhances your babies' ability to breathe on their own.

E ALERT!

Many premature babies suffer permanent lung damage due to the time spent on the ventilator and must cope with chronic lung problems throughout their lives. It is crucial that they avoid exposure to cigarette smoke after you bring them home.

Apnea, or the temporary cessation of respiration, can occur in babies born prior to thirty-four weeks and even up to thirty-six weeks. Medication can help overcome the problem. Just as a cup of coffee wakes up an adult in the morning, caffeine is used to jolt the baby's immature respiratory system back into action.

Some babies don't require a ventilator but still have trouble taking in enough air to fill their lungs. Continuous positive airway pressure (CPAP) helps accomplish that by keeping the lungs inflated via small tubes inserted into the babies' nostrils. CPAP can also be an effective transition step between the ventilator and unassisted breathing.

Cardiovascular Conditions

The heart is also profoundly affected by prematurity. Many preemie babies have heart problems. An atrial septal defect (ASD) is essentially a hole in the heart that doesn't completely close over during development. Depending on the size of the hole, the heart can still function normally, and the defect can be easily repaired without surgery when the infant is stronger. Patent ductus arteriosus (PDA) is a shunt malfunction that causes blood to divert from the lungs.

The deficiency in a preemie's lungs affects the heart also. Apnea is often accompanied by bradycardia, an abnormally low heartbeat defined as less than 60 beats per minute. If you have preemies in the NICU, you'll often hear the medical staff refer to "Aps" and "Bradys," nicknames used to describe the occurrence of apnea and bradycardia.

Neurological Impact

One of the most frightening and uncontrollable effects of premature birth is on the brain and nervous system. Unfortunately, there is little that doctors can do to treat these problems and it can be excruciating for parents to endure a "wait and see" approach.

Premature infants often suffer a variety of brain injuries. The consequences of the injuries can be mild, such as hyperactivity or learning disabilities, or much more serious, including epilepsy, cerebral palsy, mental retardation, or, ultimately, death. Fortunately, the risk of these injuries subsides after thirty-four to thirty-six weeks' gestational age.

Gastrointestinal Problems

In the womb, the placenta(s) delivered nutrients to your babies via their umbilical cords. The babies' gastrointestinal systems didn't need to take in food, digest it, derive the essential nutrients, and move it through their intestines to be excreted as waste. Once the cord is cut, however, they're out of luck. They have to take in nutrients in order to continue growing, yet their stomach and intestines aren't ready to function.

Among the many tubes and lines emanating from a preemie baby is likely to be a feeding tube to supply nutrition. These come in several forms, depending on the baby's specific feeding problems. In the most severe cases, a parenteral intravenous line bypasses the intestines to administer nutrition directly into the blood. When the stomach is able to tolerate it, the babies will be fed enterally, either through a nasogastric tube slipped through the nostrils or a tube inserted directly into the stomach through the abdominal wall. The babies' gastrointestinal systems can atrophy if not utilized, causing permanent damage, so it's important to attempt enteral feeding as soon as possible.

Unfortunately, enteral feeding has its own unpleasant consequences. Some premature infants are afflicted with a devastating gastrointestinal disorder called necrotizing enterocolitis (NEC). Essentially, tissue in the bowel dies due to infection or inflammation. It usually occurs in preemie babies about a week after birth, or after enteral feeding is initiated. In some cases, a small area of dead tissue can repair itself, but large areas of NEC will cause the bowel to rupture, allowing the septic intestinal contents to spill into the intestinal wall and eventually into the bloodstream.

Surgery can be performed to halt the progress of NEC by removing the affected portion of the intestines. In severe cases, when the entire bowel dies, transplantation is an option. In mild cases, the condition can be treated with "intestinal rest" (returning to parenteral feeding), antibiotics, and nasogastric drainage. Babies usually recover from NEC, and it does not usually produce any long-lasting gastrointestinal disorders.

Breast milk has been proven to help prevent NEC in premature babies. Even though they can't directly nurse their babies at first, mothers of multiples are strongly encouraged to provide milk by pumping their breasts.

Premature babies are also quite susceptible to constipation, and are often treated with medications, such as glycerin or laxatives, to stimulate their bowels. Because breast milk is generally gentler on premature digestive systems, providing expressed milk is one way that you can help alleviate your babies' suffering.

Delicate Skin

A premature baby does not look like a normal newborn. If you look past the tubes, contraptions, and devices surrounding them, one of the first things that you'll notice is the appearance of their skin. Discolored and shiny, it may be covered with fine downy hair, called lanugo. Babies in the watery womb don't need the same kind of protective covering that they require in an air environment, and don't develop the "thicker" skin that we're accustomed to seeing on full term infants until thirty-four to thirty-six weeks gestation.

Their thin skin and lack of body fat also inhibit a preemie's ability to regulate his body temperature. Many premature infants are housed in incubators or isolettes, clear plastic boxes, to help them keep warm. Because they create a barrier around the babies, they may feel intimidating to parents who want closer contact with their children, but they serve an important purpose in helping babies adjust to life outside the womb.

Premature skin can be very sensitive to touch. Your doctors, nurses and caretakers will advise you on how to interact most comfortably with your babies. It is frustrating and disheartening not to be able to hold and caress your eagerly awaited infants. Give them time to grow and develop, and stay focused on the time when you'll have the opportunity for closer contact.

Kangaroo care is a pleasant procedure that not only helps your baby maintain her temperature but also promotes parental bonding. Babies are positioned skin-to-skin on your chest, allowing your body heat to radiate onto them. It's a warm, cozy experience that fathers can participate in as well as mothers.

Additional Complications

Numerous other complications are associated with prematurity. Sometimes during the NICU experience, it may seem that every improvement is accompanied by one or more additional problems. Because your premature babies have missed out on crucial development time in the womb, they are being forced to adjust to life in a harsher environment, and the impact of that is manifested in many different ways. Oftentimes, the very treatments that are intended to preserve their life cause damage and further complications.

Some of the other conditions that your babies may have to contend with are

- **Jaundice:** This condition, characterized by yellow skin tone, is caused by excess bilirubin (a byproduct of red blood cells) in the blood. Preemies are more susceptible to jaundice because lower levels of bilirubin are toxic to their immature livers, meaning that they reach the level of "excess" more quickly. Jaundice is usually treated with phototherapy, a special type of light that helps to break up the bilirubin.

- **Retinopathy of prematurity (ROP):** Retinal damage to the babies' eyes may cause temporary blindness and permanent vision damage. Your preemies may have to wear glasses when they grow up and should receive follow-up care from an ophthalmologist.

- **Anemia:** Preemies develop anemia for many reasons. The deficiency of red blood cells necessary to carry oxygen throughout the body may require a transfusion to correct.

- **Reflux:** Stomach acid backs up into the digestive track, causing discomfort and vomiting. Medications can control the problem and alleviate symptoms.

Other medical issues may not be apparent until months, or even years, later. They include cerebral palsy, chronic lung disorder, learning disabilities, and hyperactivity.

Surviving an NICU Stay

It's up to the medical team to help your babies survive. But what about your survival? An NICU experience can be every bit as excruciating for parents as it is for the actual patients. Having one child in the hospital is stressful, but having two, three, or even more critically ill preemies can push parents to the edge. There are some coping strategies that make the situation more bearable, and may indirectly help your babies' progress as well.

Changing Emotions, Changing Relationships

Don't be surprised by irrational reactions or unexpected emotions. Becoming a parent of preemie multiples is a tremendously stressful ordeal.

You are likely to experience a whirlwind of feelings: frustration, anxiety, loneliness, elation, hope, despair, guilt, anger, and grief. Many mothers mourn for the loss of their "normal" pregnancy; they may feel as if they've been cheated out of the last few months. You may exhibit the classic stages of grief: denial, anger, bargaining, depression, and acceptance.

You may be surprised by how the NICU experience changes every aspect of your life. Your relationships with others may take on a new dynamic. The strain of having multiples in the NICU can take a toll on marriages, as well as relationships between family members and friends. You may feel resentful toward your friends who have "normal" pregnancies and babies. You may feel angry or want to blame your spouse. You may feel irritable with well-meaning friends and relatives who are constantly asking for updates or offering to help. You can't let your emotional state affect your care and handling of the babies, and you may be called on to make vital life-or-death decisions regarding their care.

FACT

Many hospitals assign families with preemies a social worker or advocate to guide them through the maze of medical terminology, insurance claims, and other issues. A counselor may be able to help you sort through your feelings so that you are better equipped to handle the situation.

Getting Through the Tough Times

In addition to counselors and social workers, the doctors, nurses, and staff that are responsible for caring for your babies are also an invaluable resource. Everyone has personality quirks and bad days, but for the most part you will find them as a group to be incredibly knowledgeable, caring, and responsive to your questions and requests. Don't be afraid to speak up. Ask questions. Ask for clarification if you don't understand the answer. If you forget the answer, ask again. You are your children's best advocate.

Many NICU hospitals have a support network for parents of preemies. Many of the members will be fellow parents of multiples. Talking to other parents who have experienced the NICU can be very reassuring. You'll realize that you are not alone in your journey, and that other babies have survived more severe challenges than yours. If your hospital does not have a parents' network, contact your local parents of multiples club. They are likely to have members who have experienced the challenges of an NICU stay.

Because an NICU stay can extend for weeks or even months, it's important to establish a routine. You can't spend every moment at the hospital; it's important to take breaks to relieve stress, eat healthy meals, and get plenty of rest. If you have other children at home, you'll need to spend time with them as well.

Create some structure within your day, allocating time with the babies at the hospital and time to lead your life. You can easily get burned out by worry and exhaustion if you don't. Many parents find it helpful to return to work in order to keep their mind occupied. It is not disloyal to the babies to do so.

Your spirituality may be of great comfort during your family's NICU experience. NICU nurses have observed that parents who have faith in a higher power have an easier time coping with the stress. Attending religious services, praying, talking to a clergy leader, and relying on the support of a church network may provide comfort and a sense of peace amid the crisis.

Contribute What You Can

One of the most frightening and frustrating aspects of parenting preemies is a feeling of loss of control. With doctors, nurses, and medical staff in charge of your babies, it can be difficult to determine your role. You have to get permission to even touch your own children. It can be difficult to bond with your babies under these circumstances. However, there are many ways that you can participate in your babies' care. Anything you can contribute will provide a sense of control over your situation. Medical science does not underestimate the importance of parental nurturing of preemies. Here are some things to consider, provided they are approved by your hospital's NICU policies:

- Make a tape of your voice talking, singing, or reading to the babies.

- Put up pictures of loved ones in the babies' incubators.
- Do the babies' laundry.
- Take lots of pictures of your babies. (You may not think that you'll want to remember this trying time, but you will!)
- Put stuffed animals or other comfort items in the babies' beds.

Perhaps one of the most important ways that mothers can contribute to their babies' progress is by pumping breast milk. Many NICUs have pumping facilities, or you may also want to rent or buy a pump for use elsewhere. A little breast milk is better than none; more breast milk is better. The earlier you start expressing milk and the longer you can keep it up, the better. The composition of breast milk from a mother of preemies is different than from a full-term mother. Its special properties benefit the babies in many ways, helping to prevent infection and promote growth.

As your babies progress, talk to the staff about positioning them near each other. Most hospitals require that multiples be separated in order to reduce the risks of infection and mix-up, but they may be willing to consider your requests when the babies are older and healthier. Although there is no scientific proof, some theories support the idea that multiples receive comfort and strength from the close proximity.

The Road to Home

Once your babies have stabilized and conquered some of the more acute medical challenges mentioned earlier, their main requirement will be time: time to grow and develop. NICU staff often calls babies in this phase "feeders/growers." Usually babies require hospitalization until the time of their original due date, so it could be many weeks or months until your babies are big enough and strong enough to go home with you.

Discuss the standards of release with your doctors, but in most cases each baby will have to be able to do all of the following before going home:

- Suck and swallow to take in food (some babies are allowed home with a feeding tube, however).
- Urinate and defecate (in mommy language, that's "pee and poop").
- Maintain body temperature.

In all likelihood, one of your multiples will accomplish those developmental milestones before the other(s). Doctors usually observe that the first-born multiple progresses fastest, while second-borns face more challenges and complications. With higher order multiples, the pattern continues, with the last born usually exhibiting the most problems.

Although graduating from the NICU is a joyous accomplishment, it is not the end of your journey. If you have to leave one or more babies in the hospital, it can be a rather bittersweet occasion. Your routine may become more complicated as you try to balance caring for your released multiple with visits to the hospital.

Caring for Preemies at Home

Hooray! The long-awaited moment has finally arrived, and your whole family is reunited at home. Although it is a happy occasion, some parents are surprised to discover that caring for their babies at home presents its own set of challenges. Some experience a sort of delayed depression, similar to postpartum depression.

Parents of preemies should receive instruction in infant CPR so that they are able to resuscitate their babies in the event of an emergency. The staff at the NICU should be able to recommend a training program.

Hospitals acknowledge that while they are very good at caring for babies in intensive care, they are not as effective at preparing parents to care for those babies at home. Some facilities do encourage parents to care for their babies in the hospital for a night or two before they are sent home, but not much else is offered in the way of formal training.

Some of the specialized equipment that kept your babies alive in the hospital may accompany you home. Breathing monitors sound an alert if a bout of apnea occurs. Some babies may remain unable to take in food by mouth and will require feeding tubes, while others will require oxygen tanks. Be sure that you understand how to operate and maintain any specialized equipment.

Although prematurity is a very frightening subject for parents, it's also an area of medicine associated with countless stories of miracles and hope. Advances in technology make it possible for even the tiniest of babies to survive. And despite their fragile appearance, don't underestimate the strength of premature infants, described by one neonatologist as "the strongest creatures on earth."

As happy as you are to leave the hospital environment, it won't be long before you have to schedule a round of follow-up appointments. Your babies may require follow-up care with specialists in ophthalmology, cardiology, or pulmonology, as well as occupational therapy, physical therapy, or other specialties. Transporting the babies to and from appointments can be complicated, and during such times, an extra set of hands will prove invaluable. Your babies will also need to receive regular checkups from a pediatrician. Be sure that the doctor you choose has some experience in treating children who were born prematurely and is aware of the special challenges they may face later in life.

Some families find it awkward to accept help from others when the babies return home. After weeks or months of relinquishing control to the hospital staff, they feel compelled to control the babies' care when they come home. Don't fall into the trap of denying help when you need it. Accept offers of help, but be specific in designating which forms of help are most comfortable for you. You may be wary about letting others handle the babies for fear of spreading germs and infection. Instead, ask for help with meals, errand running, and other chores so that your time is freed up to care for the babies.

Chapter 18

E Breastfeeding and Bottle Feeding

As soon as your babies are born, you'll be faced with the first of many tough parenting choices: how to fill their hungry tummies. Instinct and scientific research confirm that breastfeeding is best, yet formula marketers offer assurance that their products offer healthy convenience. With more mouths to feed, efficiency is a priority, but not at the expense of the babies' health and well-being. Ultimately, there is no right or wrong choice, only what works best for your family.

Making the Decision

To make an informed decision about feeding your multiples, it's important to understand the advantages and disadvantages of each method. Each approach naturally has benefits as well as drawbacks, not to mention its own set of outspoken supporters who will make their opinions well known to you as soon as you announce your pregnancy.

No matter what you choose, you are likely to experience opposition about your choice. Breastfeeding advocates will try to make you think you're sacrificing your babies' well-being if you give them bottles. At the other extreme, your friends, family members, and even some medical professionals may call you crazy and try to dissuade you from exclusively breastfeeding your multiples. Ultimately, you have to do what's best for your babies; that may be breastfeeding, bottle feeding, or a combination of both.

Take the opportunity during your pregnancy to research the issue. Books, including this one, magazines, and Web sites will all reveal useful factual information. Fellow parents of multiples are also a valuable resource.

ALERT!

As you talk to other mothers about their experience, ask them how they arrived at their choice and why it worked best for them. Pay particular attention to circumstances that closely resemble your own—for example, previous nursing experience (or lack of it), working or stay-at-home parents, or supertwins.

Whatever you decide during your pregnancy, leave yourself an opportunity to change your mind once the babies arrive. You simply have no way of knowing what the future holds. Ruling out one option or the other may create more difficult circumstances for you in the long run. Even the most experienced breastfeeding advocate may find it overwhelming to nurse triplets, while the most reticent may feel compelled to nurse if her premature twins would benefit from breast milk.

Breastfeeding Multiples

Many people wrongly assume that breastfeeding twins, triplets, or more is impossible. Not only is it possible, but it can be a very rewarding experience for the entire family. You might be surprised by how many mothers exclusively breastfeed their twins and, with higher order multiples becoming more commonplace, even mothers with triplets or more have great success with nursing their babies.

The Benefits of Breastfeeding

The numerous benefits of breastfeeding are undeniable. For multiples, who are often at a developmental disadvantage due to low birth weight or prematurity, being breastfed can give them a wonderful boost. Consider the following benefits:

- Nursing aids jaw, teeth, and facial development.
- Antibodies in breast milk protect infants from illness.
- Breastfed babies have fewer allergies.
- Breastfed babies have fewer ear infections.
- Studies have shown that breastfed babies have higher IQs.
- Some studies suggest that breastfed babies grow up to have less incidence of obesity and hypertension.
- The close contact between mother and babies while nursing enhances bonding and helps the babies feel secure.

Breastfeeding also benefits the mother in several ways. For example:

- Nursing after childbirth increases the level of oxytocin in the mother, stimulating the uterus to return to normal more quickly.
- Mothers who breastfeed generally lose weight more rapidly.
- There is some evidence to suggest that breastfeeding reduces the mother's risks of certain cancers.

Finally, breastfeeding brings several benefits to the family group as a whole. First and foremost, it's free! Breastfeeding can represent a substantial savings for families with multiples. A researcher at Georgetown University Medical Center estimated that families who formula feed spend approximately $400 per month for supplies and equipment. That estimate only covers one baby; double it or triple it, and the costs skyrocket. La Leche League International estimates that breastfeeding offers families with twins an approximate savings of $1,200 and 300 hours in the first year alone!

ESSENTIAL

Regardless of the final outcome, your initial attempts to nurse in the first few days after birth are extremely beneficial to your babies. Before your milk actually comes up, your body produces colostrum, sometimes called "liquid gold" because of its highly concentrated nutrients and antibodies. It helps develop the babies' gastrointestinal systems.

In addition, breast milk is readily available. There's no mixing or reheating. It doesn't require a midnight dash to the all-night market for refills when you run out. It doesn't have to be shaken or stirred. You don't have to wash and sterilize dozens of bottles, nipples, and accessories. And it's always the perfect temperature for your babies.

Your breast milk is clearly the most desirable food source for your babies. However, breastfeeding is tremendously demanding on a mother of multiples, both physically and emotionally. It will be your primary activity during the first few months of their lives, requiring most of your time and consuming nearly all of your energy. To breastfeed exclusively requires determination, commitment, and a strong support system. Realistically, it is not the right option for every mother.

Breastfeeding Twins

When breastfeeding twins, the first question to address is: together or separately? Since most mothers have two breasts, it is often convenient to nurse both babies simultaneously. It saves a great deal of time, but can be a tricky maneuver. The process of getting two babies on and off the breast sometimes requires an extra set of hands. In the beginning, you'll probably want some assistance in getting the babies arranged for nursing. A lactation consultant or maternity nurse can help while you're still in the hospital; once you are at home with the babies, enlist the help of your partner (or someone you're comfortable exposing your breasts to).

For infant twins, the football hold works well, especially for mothers who have delivered via cesarean section. This position keeps the bulk of the babies away from the tender incision site. As the twins get bigger, the parallel, or "spoons," hold is convenient, while the criss-cross and front V positions are ideal for older babies who don't require as much head support. A good supply of pillows will support the babies so that you can use your hands elsewhere.

◀ Football Hold

◀ Parallel Hold

◀ Criss-Cross Hold

◀ Front-V Hold

Once the babies are in position near your breasts, it's time for them to latch on. One at a time, brush the babies' lips with your nipple to provoke them to open their mouths wide. As soon as there is an opening, quickly bring the baby to your breast. The babies should take the entire areola into their mouths, not just the nipple tip. Their lips should be turned out and their noses should be touching the breast. (Don't worry, they can still breathe!)

The frequency and duration of breastfeeding may vary, but most full-term newborns need to nurse ten to twelve times a day during the first few weeks. If you're feeding your babies simultaneously, it helps to keep them on the same schedule. If one baby is ready to nurse, put the other on the breast at the same time, even if you have to wake him up. Some experts decry the notion of ever waking a sleeping baby, but they probably didn't have multiples!

Can my body produce enough milk for both babies?
Breastfeeding works on a supply and demand system. The more you breastfeed, the more milk your body will produce. Nursing often and allowing the babies to empty both breasts will help you establish an ample supply of milk.

Breastfeeding Triplets or More

If you have three or more babies, you obviously won't be able to nurse them all at the same time. It is still possible to nurse triplets, quadruplets, or higher; it just takes some organization and perseverance. Mothers of higher order multiples who want to breastfeed should assume that nearly all of their waking moments in the first few weeks at home will be spent with a baby or a pump at the breast.

Many moms of multiples swear by the U-shaped nursing pillows that fit around the mother's waist and help position the babies at the right level for nursing. You'll find sources for obtaining these highly recommended products in Appendix A.

Most mothers of higher order multiples find it easiest to use a rotation feeding schedule. For example, Babies A and B will nurse at the breast while Baby C receives a bottle of expressed breast milk. At the next feeding, Babies B and C are breastfed and Baby A receives a bottle. At the third feeding, Babies A and C are at the breast while Baby B takes the bottle.

Another approach is tandem breastfeeding, or feeding each baby one after the other. It requires a lot of time and patience but allows each baby to have individual time with mom, and also ensures ample milk production. Be sure to alternate breasts as each baby feeds so that both sides will produce an equal supply.

Breastfeeding Preemies

If your multiples are born prematurely, you may not have the option to breastfeed them immediately. Preemies are often born without the ability to suck and swallow like full-term infants, so nursing may be delayed until they catch up developmentally. However, you can still provide the benefits of breastfeeding by expressing your colostrum and breast milk. Whatever amount you provide will be incorporated into their feedings and will be a welcome boost to their nutritional needs.

Potential Pitfalls

If you expect that something as natural as nursing a child would come easy, you might be surprised by how difficult it can be at times. Even if you have successfully breastfed other children, you may find that nursing multiples presents some challenges. There are going to be times when you think you simply can't do it, and want to give up. Recognizing and addressing the potential pitfalls that you may encounter along the way can help you prepare to resolve any problems if they occur.

ESSENTIAL

You can also relieve the discomfort by applying cold compresses to the breasts in between nursing sessions. Bags of frozen peas work well for this purpose! Cabbage leaves also have some unknown but effective properties that alleviate breast discomfort. Try putting them inside your nursing bra.

Many mothers give up on breastfeeding before they really get started, by not giving their body time to recover from childbirth and set up for nursing. In the first few days following birth, your breasts produce colostrum, the clear, yellowish pre-milk substance that is so rich in vital nutrients for newborns. About three days later, your milk will "come in," the term used to describe the transition from colostrum to the milky bluish-white liquid. During this time, your breasts may become very full with milk. They may feel tight, uncomfortable, or even painful. It's important to remember that this is a temporary condition that usually lasts about a day, and that the best remedy is to nurse your babies or pump out the milk.

Other signs of discomfort in your breasts, such as dry, cracked nipples or soreness after the first week, may be caused when the babies aren't latched on properly, but they can also be an indication of infection. If these problems persist, talk to your doctor or lactation consultant as soon as possible; they can usually offer some solutions so that you can continue nursing your babies.

Sometimes women are tempted to forsake breastfeeding their multiples because it is too difficult to keep things straight. It's much easier to keep track of how many ounces each baby ingests when you can measure out the amount in a bottle. But remember, the mother's body will respond to her babies' demand for food; try not to worry as much about the exact quantity of intake, and concentrate more on your babies' behavior. Keep a chart to track each baby's nursing patterns. Establish a system that works for you; some mothers prefer to alternate the breast their babies feed from each time, others find that too complicated and assign each baby to the right or left side. Study and learn each baby's hunger cues, such as

- Open lips
- Sucking on fist or fingers (or their co-multiple's body parts!)
- Rooting, or turning their open mouth toward the breast
- Fretful sounds

Although most experts advocate nursing on demand, especially in the first month to establish your milk supply, with multiples it's usually easier to follow a schedule. Early on, the babies may need to nurse every two hours, for as long as twenty minutes a session, especially since even full-term twins or multiples tend to be smaller birth weights. As they grow, the schedule will expand to every three or four hours. You'll know your babies are receiving sufficient nutrition by their output. Talk to your doctor or lactation consultant about what to look for in the first week, as stool frequency and appearance will differ from day to day and from baby to baby. After the first week, your babies should have at least six wet diapers and usually one soiled diaper per day. With more than one baby, don't rely on memory. Use a chart or log (see Appendix B for a sample) to help you keep track of who did what and when. If your babies exhibit any of the symptoms listed below, talk to your pediatrician, nurse, or lactation consultant to ensure that they are not dehydrated or malnourished.

- Listlessness, with a weak cry
- Sunken spot on the top of the head
- Dry lips
- Discoloration or yellowing of the skin, or skin that doesn't spring back when lightly pinched

Finally, the emotional and psychological burdens of breastfeeding multiples can discourage a mother from breastfeeding. There's simply no private and discreet way to nurse two babies simultaneously, making it difficult to breastfeed them in public. It can be frustrating to be confined at home with little else to do but feed babies all day and night.

ALERT!

Sometimes breastfeeding can be an issue of dissension between couples, especially if the mother's partner resents the breasts' functional change from sexual to nutritional. Open and honest communication about the issue, beginning during the pregnancy, will help you work through the problem.

Any of these potential pitfalls, as well as a slew of others not mentioned here, may prompt you to abandon breastfeeding. It's important to make the decision with careful consideration, not in the midst of a hormone-crazed and sleep-deprived haze. Organize a support network that you can call on in times of trouble, including experienced mothers of multiples, your pediatrician, your lactation consultant, and trusted friends. They will assist you through the rough times, remind you of your commitment to give your babies the best possible start in life, and keep you on the path to breastfeeding success.

Getting the Right Nutrients

One of the biggest factors influencing the outcome of breastfeeding is maternal health. Just like a factory that relies on sufficient resources to manufacture products, the nursing mother's body requires proper caloric and fluid intake, as well as a nutritionally balanced diet, to produce breast milk. Remember, what goes into your mouth will be passed along to your babies via your milk. Just as in pregnancy, your health and well-being is of utmost priority while breastfeeding.

Throughout your pregnancy, your body experienced tremendous changes, including weight gain. After delivery, some of the extra pounds may decide to stick around. As tempting as it is to try to shed them immediately, restricting your diet while breastfeeding is not a wise approach. Fortunately, an added benefit of breastfeeding is that it utilizes some of the stored fat on your body, helping you to lose weight!

If you're trying to produce milk for two, three, or more babies, you'll have to eat enough to compensate. Experts recommend adding about 500 extra calories to your normal pre-pregnancy diet, approximately the amount found in a peanut butter sandwich or a cup of ice cream, but that's just for one baby! You'll have to adjust accordingly depending on how many babies you're feeding.

A healthful breastfeeding diet is more than just eating extra food. What food you eat has a big impact on the quality of the breast milk that you produce. Choose foods with nutritional power, not the empty calories of junk food. Good choices for a breastfeeding diet are

- Lean meats
- High-fiber whole grain cereals and breads
- Fresh fruit or 100% fruit juices
- Colorful vegetables, especially leafy greens
- Low-fat cheese or yogurt
- Eggs
- Beans

In addition to eating enough, you've also got to drink! It's much easier for your body to make milk if it's fueled with lots of liquids. Water is always the best choice, but juices and milk are good options also. You can also eat hydrating foods like fruits and soups. However, avoid caffeinated and alcoholic drinks. You don't want to pass along the effects of those drinks to the babies.

One way to ensure that you take in ample fluids is to drink a glass of water before beginning a nursing session. Then, refill the glass and keep it within reach so you can sip it while you breastfeed.

Sometimes certain foods the mother consumes can cause distress for the babies. Foods that cause gas, heartburn, or other digestive reactions for you will likely have the same effect on the babies, so avoid them while you're nursing. It takes about six hours for what you've eaten to have an impact on the composition of your breast milk. If you notice that a particular food item aggravates one or more of the babies, resulting in excess gas, spitting up, or fussiness, you'll want to stay away from that food until you have completed breastfeeding and weaned the babies.

Alternative Feeding Using Breast Milk

Despite your best intentions, it may not be possible to immediately nurse your multiples in the traditional way. If you want to be sure that they receive all the benefits of breast milk, but are restricted from breastfeeding, there are some alternative methods you can employ.

Supplemental Nutrition Systems

For some families, certain conditions may prohibit one or all of the babies from breastfeeding normally. As mentioned earlier, premature babies often haven't developed a sufficient sucking reflex. Or perhaps a baby's deformity, such as cleft palate, prevents nursing. Sometimes a mother is restricted from breastfeeding, either temporarily or permanently, but still wishes to pass along the benefits of breast milk. For any of these situations, devices exist that will allow you to simulate the experience of breastfeeding.

Finger feeding is an alternative method generally employed for short-term delivery of breast milk to a baby that is unable to nurse. The baby sucks on a tube attached to an adult's finger. Finger feeding can be instrumental in helping a baby develop proper nursing skills and also provides the intimacy of skin-to-skin contact.

A supplemental nursing system (SNS) delivers breast milk from a bottle via a tube connected to the mother's breast. A bottle containing breast milk hangs from the mother's neck, with tiny soft tubes that are taped to her breast, ending right at her nipple. The baby latches on to the mother's breast, including the tube, and receives milk just as if he were nursing.

Many adoptive mothers have been able to breastfeed babies using a SNS. The effect of the baby's nursing stimulates the hormone prolactin and can actually induce lactation even though the mother was never pregnant.

Pumping

For moms of preemies or higher order multiples, pumping breast milk is a necessity; even mothers of full-term twins will find it to be a benefit. Expressing milk in the first few weeks enhances the supply of milk, ensuring that there is enough to go around. Meanwhile, building a stored surplus of expressed milk may also prove beneficial if mom needs a break—for example, if she is returning to work or wants to give dad a chance to feed the babies.

Breast pumps are available in two formats: hand-operated and electric or battery-operated. Hand pumps are useful for initial expressing of milk to establish supply in the first few weeks, but won't be very helpful for the mother who wishes to collect milk in greater quantities. The more powerful electric pumps are required for that job. You can buy a pump at any baby supply store, but might want to consider renting one. You'll get a top-quality piece of equipment designed for frequent use, and it may save you some money.

E
ALERT!

Whatever equipment you use, be sure to select a product with double suction cups that allow you to pump both breasts simultaneously. It's a tremendous timesaver and regulates milk production equally on both sides so that you don't end up lopsided!

To ensure a successful pumping session, follow these guidelines:

- Drink a glass of water before starting.
- Sit down in a comfortable, peaceful location.
- Look at your babies or a picture of your babies to encourage let-down of your milk.
- Use the proper collection receptacle for your breast pump model.
- Label the expressed milk and store it properly immediately after it is collected.

Breast milk should be refrigerated unless it is going to be used immediately. Refrigerated milk should be consumed within a week, but it will keep in the freezer for months.

Bottle Feeding

There are many reasons why families with multiples elect to bottle feed their babies. It definitely offers several advantages over breastfeeding, most notably that it allows someone other than the mother to be the primary source of food. Modern infant formulas, while not as perfectly nutritionally sound as breast milk, are able to provide a healthy alternative with the convenience of bottle delivery.

Bottle feeding requires a stockpile of supplies, and when there's more than one baby, all of the bottles, nipples, and formula may fill an entire pantry! It's always good to keep plenty on hand—running out when you have two or more hungry infants is not an option.

Before you leave the hospital, your pediatrician should advise you about the type of formula to feed your babies. Usually an iron-fortified product made from cow's milk is recommended for newborns, because it most closely simulates human breast milk. However, your doctor may recommend other products, such as soy formula for lactose intolerance or hypoallergenic products for allergy-prone babies. Don't give your baby alternative products unless instructed by your doctor.

FACT

If your babies require different types of formula, you can keep things straight by color-coding their bottles. Either buy different colors or use a permanent marker to make an identifying mark.

Formula Basics

Formula comes in two basic forms. The most convenient—and most expensive—formulas are ready-to-eat. Some even come in their own disposable bottles! Others need to be dispensed into bottles. It's usually more cost-effective to use a formula product in a concentrated or powdered form; these are mixed with water before being served to the babies.

Some experts recommend sterilizing the water used for formula destined for infants under six months of age. Boiling the water removes impurities and kills potentially harmful bacteria. You may find it easier to skip that step and instead purchase bottled water. Discuss your local water supply conditions with your doctor to help you decide what's best for your babies.

You may be puzzled by the diverse brands of formula on the market. The U.S. Food and Drug Administration (FDA) regulates the manufacture of infant formula to ensure that it is safe and nutritious. Both generic and brand-name products have to meet these federal standards. To your babies, the difference between one brand and the other can be equated to an adult's preference for Coke or Pepsi: a matter of taste. If you have a strong preference for one, you may find the alternative unacceptable. Likewise, your babies may protest if you switch products on them!

QUESTION?

Our water comes from a well. Is it safe to use in formula for the babies?
Well water often has a high concentration of contaminants and nitrates. Boiling it only increases the concentration of those elements. You should consider using bottled water for your babies' formula.

Bottle Basics

Many bottle-feeding systems are available, and all have their own unique features. Ultimately, the best product is the one that works best for you and your family. Younger infants will need smaller four- or six-ounce bottles with low-flow nipple holes. As the babies grow, however, a feeding may average more than eight ounces, requiring larger bottles and nipples that allow a faster delivery of formula. You'll need at least one bottle per baby, but it's much more convenient to have a surplus.

Nipples are available in a wide range of styles, and it may take some experimentation to find the ones that work best for your babies. Some nipple styles mimic breastfeeding, and are designed to reduce nipple confusion for mothers who choose to combine bottle feeding with nursing. Orthodontic nipples are shaped to properly develop a baby's gums and palate. Other nipple styles restrict the amount of air that babies intake as they suck formula, reducing (in theory, anyway) the discomfort of a gassy tummy.

ALERT!

It may be helpful to mix up formula in big batches to last throughout an entire day. Mix up enough to last several feedings in a large pitcher that you can keep in the refrigerator until needed. Or, dispense your batch of formula into bottles that are ready when the babies are hungry.

There's no physical reason why babies require a warm bottle, but some do prefer it that way. Room temperature formula is usually comfortable for most babies, but since some formula products require refrigeration, you may find it necessary to warm up bottles before serving. If you choose to heat bottles, keep in mind that breast milk is delivered at body temperature, 98.6

degrees. Formula should never be served any hotter! Microwaving bottles is not recommended, since the liquid can heat unevenly. Despite that fact, many parents still do it. If you choose to, proceed cautiously. Always shake microwaved bottles thoroughly to disperse the heat, and test the contents to ensure they won't burn your babies' tender mouths.

To be safe rather than sorry, simply set the bottles in a pan of hot tap water for a few minutes to warm them. Electric bottle warmers are another option; they're probably not worth the cost for just one baby, but come in handy when you're warming multiple bottles.

Position Points

Proper positioning of the babies for feeding is important whether you are breastfeeding or bottle feeding. Be sure to support the babies' heads and bodies securely. Refer to the diagrams for nursing positions earlier in this chapter and emulate them for bottle feeding; the close contact and intimacy is important for bonding. Alternate sides and direction to enhance the babies' visual and cognitive development. Finally, holding a baby in a semi-upright position with the bottle at an angle helps prevent air intake.

Although it's tempting, and sometimes a matter of necessity, bottle propping is discouraged. Instead, consider a hands-free bottle, like the Podee products, for those times when you have more babies than hands. These bottles allow the container to rest upright by funneling the fluid into the nipple via a tube. It won't be long before the babies will be able to hold their bottles themselves! In the meantime, your infants should be held as much as possible during feedings. Use the time to cuddle and coo; make eye contact.

Combination Approach

Some families find that a combination of breast and bottle works best for feeding their babies, as this offers the advantages of both methods. Alternating between nursing and giving a bottle of either formula or expressed breast milk allows fathers and helpers an opportunity to feed a baby and gives mom a much-needed break. Each family has to find the system that best meets their needs. There are several ways to combine approaches:

- **Alternate babies:** One gets the breast, the other gets the bottle, and they switch at the next feeding.
- **Alternate feedings:** Breastfeed all babies one time, bottle feed the next.
- **Day/night rotation:** Breastfeed during the day, bottle feed at night. Alternately, working moms might try the opposite approach.
- **As needed:** Primarily breastfeed, but supplement with a bottle when mom needs a break.

Nipple confusion can be a concern when you combine the bottle and the breast. Sometimes babies prefer the relative ease of bottle feeding over a breastfeeding session where they have to work a little harder to suck milk. Other babies may prefer the closeness and comfort of breastfeeding and refuse to take a bottle if mom is nearby.

Whatever works for your family is the best option. Don't be swayed by well-intentioned but misguided advice from others. Have confidence in your ability to parent your multiples and to make the right feeding choices. Together, you and your babies will establish a routine that delivers optimum nutrition and convenience.

Chapter 19

The First Few Months

Introducing twins, triplets, or more into a family demands some adjustment from everyone involved. The new babies are getting used to breathing, eating, and sleeping. The parents are juggling their work and home responsibilities while trying to meet the needs of two or more infants. Older siblings have to get used to sharing the spotlight with the new additions. Even the family pet has to adjust to the new smells, sounds, and schedules.

Getting Sleep

What's the hardest thing about having newborn multiples? Ask any parent, and you'll likely hear a common lament: lack of sleep. With babies that need to eat every two to three hours around the clock, parents' normal nighttime sleep routine is out the window. Rather than retiring at 10:00 P.M. and rising refreshed at 7:00 A.M., they find themselves dozing for an hour in between feedings at 3:00 A.M., and catching a catnap at 3:00 P.M.

How Babies Sleep

Newborns need a lot of sleep. Unfortunately, the sleep patterns of young infants aren't concentrated during the nighttime hours, like adults'. Throughout a twenty-four hour cycle, babies sleep, wake up to eat, and return to sleep several times. As they grow older, they'll start to extend the amount of time between feedings, and thus stay asleep for longer periods of time. But in the meantime, parents have to adjust to a schedule of sleeping in short intervals.

Most full-term, normal birth weight newborns require between sixteen and eighteen hours of sleep a day. During the first few weeks, that time is spread throughout the day and night, in two- to three-hour bursts. Singleton parents can focus their attention on the baby when he awakes, then return to sleep when he does. The challenge for parents of multiples is that their babies' sleep patterns may not coincide, greatly reducing the amount of available rest periods in between feedings. In addition, multiples tend to be smaller; they often need to eat more frequently, and it may take more time for them to develop the ability to stay asleep for longer intervals.

Babies' sleep needs vary greatly. Some are able to stay asleep for five or six hours at a stretch as young as six weeks old. Others may take six months before they can sleep this long. There is no way to anticipate when that particular milestone will occur for each of your multiples; just rest assured that it will happen eventually.

Coping with the Lack of Sleep

So you've accepted the fact that having newborn multiples is going to be physically exhausting at times. There are some strategies that will help you survive the trying time until you can catch up on sleep.

Remember that infancy is temporary and fleeting. Your babies will grow older and stronger and they WILL sleep through the night. Rest assured that the day will eventually arrive, and take comfort in realizing that every new dawn brings you one day closer to that milestone.

From the very beginning, establish healthy sleep habits for your babies. The cozy, dark environment of the womb didn't distinguish between night and day, so newborns need some time to adjust to the new schedule. Many are born with their days and nights mixed up, being most alert in the middle of the night and sleeping soundly throughout the day. To encourage them to learn the difference, you can stimulate their senses when they are awake during the day, and keep things still and quiet at night. For example, use bright lights, background music, and a cheerful voice during daytime feedings, but keep the lights dim and your voice low at night.

Swaddling, the practice of wrapping babies "burrito style" in soft blankets, is comforting to many babies and may help them to feel snug and secure while sleeping. It's most commonly used with newborns who are still accustomed to the close confines of their mother's womb. Research has shown that swaddled babies sleep more deeply and fall back asleep more readily when awakened. It's also been proven to reduce the risk of sudden infant death syndrome (SIDS) because it keeps babies in the safest position, sleeping on their backs. Babies usually outgrow the comforting effects of swaddling after a month or two.

Some families find it helpful to take a tag-team approach in order to provide each parent with an opportunity for uninterrupted sleep. Mom might take the 9:00 P.M. to 2:00 A.M. shift, then Dad takes over until the morning. If you have access to helpers, whether hired or willing volunteers, make the most of their assistance while you catch up on rest.

Finally, make resting a priority. Napping can be restorative when you can't get a full night's sleep. Sleep when the babies sleep; don't try to use that time to catch up on other things. Housework can wait!

Don't allow young infants to sleep through their feedings during the first week or so, especially if they were born early. They need consistent nutrition in order to grow and develop. It may seem like a blessing, but sleeping for more than five hours at a stretch during the first few weeks may actually be a sign of a weakened state or even dehydration.

Setting Schedules

Probably the most effective way to maximize your sleep opportunities is to get your babies on the same schedule. If you can feed them all at the same time, and get them to sleep at the same time, then you've won the game. Because every infant is an individual, that is not always possible, but it is reasonable to establish a schedule that works out most of the time.

Feeding Schedules

Ideally, feeding on demand is the recommended approach for nurturing a singleton newborn. However, most parents of multiples find that it is more efficient to implement a more scheduled routine. That's not to say that you should ignore your babies' cues. You should never deny food to a hungry baby or ignore a baby's cries. Rather, you can gently encourage the babies to follow a complementary schedule by putting them to sleep together, changing diapers at the same time, and initiating simultaneous feedings.

Your schedule should be an organic plan that is constantly updated to meet your babies' changing needs, as well as the rest of the family's activities. You may encounter times when the babies appear to be hungrier more frequently. This behavior often precedes a growth spurt. During this enhanced period of growth and development, you'll need to adapt your schedule to meet their demand.

Growth spurts are good! They usually come before a period of increased sleeping. They frequently occur at about two weeks, six weeks, three months, and six months, but babies' timetables vary greatly.

Other Routines

Establishing a routine for other activities in your day will help keep the family organized and on track. The consistency provides a sense of security for your babies, because they know what to expect. For example, give the babies a bath at about the same time each day. As much as possible, schedule outings and errands during a designated time.

Easing your babies into a sleep routine will also help them to sleep longer and more soundly. Don't expect them to follow a sleep routine immediately, however. It will take some time to establish an acceptable routine, as the babies develop the ability to sleep for longer stretches at a time and concentrate their sleep hours overnight. But it's never too early to start constructing bedtime routines, using patterns of behavior that cue the babies that it's time to sleep. For example, an evening routine of a bath, followed by a feeding and snuggle time before putting each baby in his or her crib can help the babies recognize bedtime.

Baby Care Multiplied

Leaving the hospital with the babies can be a terrifying event for new parents of multiples. With two or more tiny newborns dependent on you for their every need, it's no wonder if you feel anxious and overwhelmed! Don't let yourself worry too much—despite their fragile appearance, newborns are actually quite sturdy little creatures. Take confidence in your ability to parent your new multiples. With a little bit of creativity and organization, you'll be able to manage just fine.

For the first few months, your job is to keep the babies fed, clean, and clothed. That's not so hard, right? The challenge in caring for multiples is that they often have the same needs simultaneously, and you've only got two hands.

To keep your hands free, a baby carrier can be a lifesaver. Backpacks and front packs are great for babies who can hold their head up, but not very effective for newborns. A sling style carrier is a better option for newborns. Another option is to utilize the infant carriers that coordinate with your car seats. They make a comfortable resting place for the babies and are easy to transport through the house. Bouncy seats are another inexpensive type of equipment that fulfills this role.

Bathing Basics

Because bathing a baby takes at least two hands, it's best to bathe multiples one at a time. This means bath time is one time where you can really make use of any available help. Fortunately, newborns don't get very dirty, so they only require a full bath a few times a week.

Perhaps the easiest approach is to set up bouncy seats or infant carriers in the bathroom or near the sink where you will bathe the babies. (It's easiest to bathe young infants in a sink or basin rather than a bathtub. You only need to use a couple of inches of water and it will be easier to maintain a firm grip on their slippery skin within the confines of a smaller space.) Have all supplies ready and within arm's reach: soap, shampoo, washcloths, towels (plenty of them!), and diapers. Put the babies in their seats as you ready the water.

ALERT!

Always fill the tub and test the temperature before you place a baby in the water. Never leave an infant in a tub while the water is running. The flowing water could change temperature and scald the baby's tender skin.

As you bathe the first baby, the other multiple(s) can remain in their seats. They are safely within your sight and will be comforted by the sound of your voice. If you have older children, they can be extremely helpful during this time, by passing supplies and entertaining the waiting babies. They will enjoy participating in the babies' care, and you'll appreciate the extra set of hands, even if they are small! After you bathe and dry the first baby, he can be returned (with luck, content and soothed after the bath!) to his seat while you attend to his brothers or sisters.

Once your babies are a little bit older, you can bathe them in the bathtub using specially secured baby bath seats. One of the great joys of having multiple infants is watching the fun as they interact in the tub, splashing and enjoying the water. Of course, you should never leave babies unattended in the tub, even for a moment.

Changing Challenges

You'll do lots of changing in the first few months with multiples . . . changing diapers, changing clothes, and changing diapers again! As you get acquainted with your babies' individual habits, you'll figure out a system that works best for your family. Most families with multiples find that it saves time to change everyone together. If one is dirty, it's likely the other(s) will be too, and if not, they will be soon enough!

Diaper time is an excellent time to attend to your newborns' special needs. If your male multiples have been circumcised, you may be advised to change the dressing on their penis. Use small gauze strips and antibacterial ointment to cover the affected area until it heals, according to your doctor's instructions.

In the United States, about 65 percent of newborn boys are circumcised at birth. Circumcision is usually performed by your obstetrician in the hospital, but only on healthy babies. The procedure may be delayed if a baby is born prematurely or if there are other complications.

For boys and girls, the umbilical cord stump should be checked daily. The remains of the cord that connected the baby's belly button to the placenta will dry up and fall off within about two weeks after birth. You should not try to remove it. At your doctor's suggestion, you can clean it gently by wiping around the base with a cotton swab dipped in alcohol. However, you may be instructed to leave the area alone, under the premise that it will heal faster on its own. Keep the area dry and protected from irritation from diapers or constricted clothing.

Dressing Multiples Alike

The issue of coordinated dressing is a hot topic among parents. Some find it a cute and fun aspect of having multiples. Others believe that it detracts from their children's individuality. No research exists to confirm that the practice is damaging to multiples' sense of self, but you should be sensitive to your children's feelings about the issue once they're old enough to express a preference. In the meantime, your babies won't care as long as their clothes are comfortable and cozy, so take advantage of their infancy to dress them up to your heart's content.

Duplicate outfits can be a curse or a convenience; it's certainly easier to tell twins apart when they're dressed differently. However, when you're overwhelmed with the day-to-day details of caring for twin infants, it's much simpler to choose one outfit rather than two.

If you're conflicted about the issue, consider a compromise. Save the matching outfits for photo opportunities or special occasions. Use coordinated or similar outfits, rather than exact matches, to experience the fun without creating a cookie-cutter effect. Or assign each multiple a color, and then choose clothing (and later, toys, sippy cups, and everything else!) to match. Not only does it help to identify the individual child, but it makes it much easier to settle ownership disputes when they reach the age of such squabbles.

Crying Is Communicating

Newborn babies are a feast for the senses: the sight of ten perfect tiny toes, the smell of their tender skin, the silky softness of their downy hair. One of the great joys of having multiples is being able to revel in these glorious sensations. However, the sound of multiple newborns is not always quite so pleasant for parents. Newborn babies cry, and when you have multiples, it can sound like a never-ending cacophony.

Researchers estimate that babies spend one to two hours a day crying. Multiply that by two for twins or three for triplets, and that's an awful lot of bawling!

Interpreting the Cries

Imagine if your babies were born with the ability to say, "Hi, Mom and Dad! We love our new home, but isn't it about time for dinner?" Unfortunately, language is an acquired skill, and until it develops, babies have to rely on other forms of communication.

Their primary mode is crying. If you think about crying as communication rather than as an annoying emission of useless sound, you'll be a much more effective—and much less frustrated—parent. It's your job to translate the cries and craft an appropriate response.

Babies cry for many reasons. They may be hungry and need to be fed. They may have a dirty diaper and need to be changed. They may be too warm or too cold. In addition to physical needs, they may also cry as a reaction to emotional needs, such as when they are overstimulated, startled, or seeking the comforting touch of a loving parent.

As you get to know your newborns, you'll learn to interpret their cries more effectively. Simply spending time with each baby will help you understand their language of crying. Through trial and error you'll learn how to satisfy their needs. External cues may also be helpful in interpreting their cries. A baby who is crying because she is tired may yawn, while a hungry baby may gnaw on her fist. An unusually loud or high-pitched cry may indicate illness or pain.

ESSENTIAL

The WhyCry baby crying analyzer claims to have a 98 percent success rate in interpreting a baby's cries and letting parents know whether the baby is hungry, bored, uncomfortable, sleepy, or stressed. This system includes a monitor that digitally analyzes changes in the baby's cry frequency, pitch, and volume.

With multiples, you'll face the additional challenge of distinguishing the individual cries of each baby. Even as newborns, your multiples are unique individuals. Each has his own needs and his own style of expressing them. It's important to respond to them as individuals, rather than always as a group.

Coping with Crying

Crying is a part of life when you're caring for babies. Unfortunately, it can often become a source of frustration. As a parent, you want so badly to be able to soothe and comfort your children, and inconsolable crying may feel like a failure of that goal.

When the crying becomes overwhelming, it's vital that you take steps to avoid losing control. There will be times when all the babies are crying at the same time, and you simply aren't able to stop it. When that happens, try one of these coping strategies:

- Walk away. Put the babies in a safe, secure place, such as a crib or playpen, and walk into another room for a minute. Take deep breaths to calm down. Count to twenty and then return to the babies.
- Use a calm, soothing voice to talk to the babies. It doesn't matter what you say. The sound of your voice may offer some temporary consolation, or at the very least, reassure them that you are aware of their needs.
- If their crying escalates over your calm voice, try singing! It may not stop the crying, but it will distract you from the chaos at hand and help you endure the maelstrom.

Above all, keep a sense of humor. In a few years, this will be a funny memory of life with multiples!

Keeping Things Straight

With more than one baby in the house, it can be tough to keep track of all the details. Who ate what and when and how much? Was it Twin A who had a dirty diaper this morning or Twin B? Did you give all three babies their medicines or did someone get a double dose? Staying organized and having a system for record-keeping are important skills for new parents of multiples.

With your brain befuddled by lack of sleep, your first task is to remember which baby is which. If your multiples are identical, that can be tricky. Even dizygotic multiples can have remarkably similar appearances as newborns. The first step in keeping things straight is to make each baby easily identifiable at first glance. Some parents find it helpful to dress each multiple in a designated color. If color coordinating their wardrobe seems too complicated, consider other apparel clues: distinguishing hats, booties, or pacifier clips.

There's one downside to color-coding; eventually your babies will get undressed! If you rely too steadily on clothing cues, you'll likely become very confused when they're naked, for example, at bath time. Just in case, you can paint one tiny toe with a small dab of nail polish as a hint.

Many parents of monozygotic—or identical—twins worry that they won't be able to tell their twosome apart. Veteran parents, however, acknowledge that it's not as difficult as you would think. Even though identical twins have similar physical appearances, those that know them intimately will have no trouble distinguishing them. There are exceptions, of course. Everyone gets mixed up occasionally when they are bleary-eyed from lack of sleep!

Once you can easily identify each baby, you'll need an organized system of tracking their vital information. Many parents rely on a chart similar to that found in Appendix B. During the first weeks at home, it's vital to track crucial information about the babies' intake and output. If you are establishing breastfeeding, you'll want to keep track of how long each baby fed, and which breast they fed from. If you are combining breast milk and formula, a chart is very handy for keeping track of the alternating feedings. As gross as it sounds, monitoring the babies' diaper debris can help you ensure that they are getting proper nutrition and that their brand-new digestive systems are functioning properly. This is another instance where a chart or written record comes in very handy. Find a process that works for your family. You want a system that allows you to record important information without becoming cumbersome or an inconvenient burden.

Bonding with Everyone

When you're a parent of multiples, you become very invested in ensuring that each child receives his or her "fair share." You expend a lot of energy trying to keep things equal. Many expectant parents of multiples express concern that they won't be able to bond equally with each child. Will they have enough love to go around? Fortunately, the reality of having multiples is that a parent's capacity to love only increases exponentially in proportion to the number of children. Multiples only multiply the amount of love in a family, they don't divide it!

What Is Bonding?

Modern parents put a lot of emphasis on the process of bonding with their babies. The term describes the intense attachment that forms between parent and child. In a nutshell, it's like falling in love with your baby. In the short term, it provides the motivation for parents to fulfill their child's needs, even at the sacrifice of their own. Over the long term, effective parent-child bonding is credited with numerous influences in a child's development. It provides the model for the child's future intimate relationships. It fosters a sense of security for the child and is said to enhance self-esteem.

FACT

The process of bonding with babies was first defined in the 1970s by two professors of pediatrics, Dr. Marshall Klaus and Dr. John Kennell. Their research changed the way that hospitals handle babies immediately following birth, encouraging them to give mothers and babies time together to bond.

Sometimes bonding occurs instantaneously after birth, but for other families, it develops over time with routine caregiving. Sometimes the process is interrupted—for example, in situations where parents and child are separated shortly after birth, perhaps by a medical event. Such is frequently the case with multiples, many of whom are born prematurely or with other medical concerns. However, these impediments should not diminish bonding if parents are determined to overcome them.

Bonding with More Than One

There are many ways that parents of multiples can enhance their bond with their children. The strengthening of the emotional connection between parent and infant is accomplished by touch and smell. As much as circumstances permit, spend time holding and cuddling each baby individually.

Face-to-face interaction is also important; look into your babies' eyes at every opportunity. Any of the following activities may be helpful in enhancing bonding. Take turns with each baby.

- Infant massage or other loving touch
- Singing
- Reading (it's never to early to start!)
- Skin-to-skin contact
- Rocking
- Talking and playing

It's not uncommon for parents to occasionally feel more attached to one baby. There's nothing wrong with that, as long as the feelings of attachment do not cause you to neglect the other multiple(s). Most parents find that feelings of partiality alternate among the children over time. If you are feeling an enduring preference for one multiple, you can overcome it by consciously spending more time with the other baby or babies.

Getting Out and About

Once you've mastered the routines at home, it's time to venture out into the world. You can't stay in the house forever! Getting out and about with infant multiples can be quite a challenge, requiring the planning skills of an army general, the packing power of a mule, and the arms of an octopus. There's no need to become a hermit, however. Some simple strategies will make on-the-go maneuvering more manageable.

The first requirement for heading out is a good stroller. You'll find that your investment in a quality double, triple, or quadruple stroller pays off the first time you leave the house. With newborns, you may need to adapt the stroller to accommodate their "floppy" bodies. If your model adjusts, fold down the seats to form an open carriage and lay the babies in the space. Or prop up the babies in their seats using rolled-up blankets or head rests to support their necks. (Chapter 10 includes lots of information to help you choose the right stroller.)

If you're traveling by car, it's imperative that your vehicle is equipped with approved infant car seats—one for each baby. In most states, the law requires that infants under twenty pounds be seated in the back seat in a rear-facing seat. Be sure that your car seats are properly installed. The make and model of your vehicle will determine the best arrangement of the seats within the car. Some cars are not wide enough to accommodate three seats across, so if you have triplets, or twins and an older child, you may have to consider other options and invest in a new vehicle.

ALERT!

Before you head out for the first time, confirm your plans with your babies' doctor. Don't risk exposure to germs if your babies are still recovering from prematurity or are especially susceptible to illness, and stay home if the weather is particularly nasty.

Carrying Case: The Diaper Bag

A diaper bag is a standard accompaniment for any family on the go with a baby, but what if you have multiples? You'll want to stock your bag with plenty of supplies, but you don't necessarily need to double or triple up. You will need a larger bag, however. Alternative bag styles might be a better option when you have twins or more. Consider a backpack or a larger tote.

In addition to diaper supplies, carry an extra outfit for each baby and feeding supplies (if you'll be out during mealtime). If your babies are partial to pacifiers, make sure you stash extras, and that you have enough to go around. A portable pad or blanket is a handy addition as well, providing a sanitary spot for changes when facilities aren't available on the go. Bibs, burp rags, plastic bags, and antibacterial hand sanitizer will be very helpful for cleanups. You don't want your bag to become burdensome to carry, but other handy items you might include are: bottled water, toys (rattles, teething rings, or small books), medications, and an extra shirt for mom, just in case.

Always keep your diaper bag packed and ready to go. Restock items that you've depleted as soon as you return home, so that you don't have to rush around the next time you're trying to get out the door.

You may find it easier to have help the first few times you venture out. Often the first outing is to the pediatrician for a checkup, which can be a stressful experience in itself. You'll appreciate having an extra pair of hands available until you're comfortable juggling all the babies and their supplies on your own.

Chapter 20

Special Situations

Every set of multiples joins a unique family, with its own special routines, challenges, and relationship dynamics. Sometimes special family circumstances present extra factors to consider as you prepare for the arrival of your multiples. No matter how your family is set up, adding multiples will mean a great deal of additional joy and love.

First-Time Parents

Here you are, new to parenting, and right off the bat you're being handed a double (or triple) whammy! Take heart. In some ways, having multiples first makes it easier on parents. With no previous parenting experience, you have no idea what to expect from one baby, much less two, three, or more. That's the good news; it's one situation where ignorance is definitely bliss! The bad news is that you have no previous experience. You haven't had the chance to develop confidence in your parenting instincts, or the opportunity to create timesaving routines and shortcuts. You don't yet know your strengths and weaknesses as a parent, and your relationship with your partner has not been tested by the trials of sharing responsibility for a child. You won't have the luxury of adapting gradually to your expanded family, but will have to jump right in with both hands and both feet.

Getting Ready

With no other children at home, you have no excuse not to take it easy during your pregnancy. Use that time to read about and research parenting and pregnancy; with no prior pregnancy as a basis for comparison, you're less likely to know when something's out of the ordinary.

You have a lot more work to do in preparing your home to accommodate babies and children. With no hand-me-downs recycled from older siblings, you're starting from scratch. You'll have to spend some time—and money—to acquire all the necessary equipment and supplies.

ALERT!

Don't feel that you have to buy out the baby supply store right away. Consult other parents for a realistic determination of what's essential immediately after the babies are born and what can wait until later on.

Adjusting to Parenthood

Upon being diagnosed with multiples, you may feel that the intensity of your pregnancy has been ratcheted up a notch. You may feel not "normal."

As you reset your expectations for the future, you may even mourn the loss of normalcy. Now that you are having twins or more, your experience may be vastly different from your friends' pregnancies and you may feel that they can't relate to you.

As a first-time parent, it's even more important that you seek out the support and advice of other parents of multiples. A local multiples group is an invaluable resource for new parents, providing mentorship and companionship. It's also crucial that you line up a helpful support system. If you don't have an established network of babysitters and health-care providers, start rounding them up well in advance of the babies' arrival. You're going to need the help!

It's easy for first-time parents to underestimate the need for assistance. You may think that you can go it alone, or that you can handle it. Maybe you feel that you don't want to impose on the friends and relatives who offer to help out. Don't turn them down just yet! Ask the parents who've lived it before you; most all will agree that they wish they had accepted more offers of help.

FACT

Having multiples can put a strain on your marriage. Thirty-nine percent of single parents of multiples reported that the emotional stress of having multiples contributed to the breakup of their marriage.

As new partners in parenthood, be gentle with your spouse through this experience. It's new for both of you, and you'll both have to adjust to new roles. The lines of responsibility are not yet clearly delineated; open communication about your expectations and your feelings will help you establish routines and a comfortable pattern of family life. All aspects of your life and your relationship will undergo a change with the arrival of these babies. Be flexible and accommodating. Support and nurture each other through the experience.

Take Heart

Above all, don't be discouraged. One of the biggest things you lack as a first-time parent is perspective. You can't see the light at the end of the tunnel. You don't know from experience that eventually the upheaval will settle into a routine. Soon enough the babies will sleep through the night, feed themselves, and leave you for part of the day to attend school. There will be a time when you'll be able once again to sleep soundly, sit down for an entire meal, and enjoy sex.

Probably the biggest surprise in store for you is the amazing wonderment of becoming a parent. You won't believe how lucky you feel to have received the gift of multiples. Just one child is a wonderful blessing. You've been gifted with the miracle of multiples. For you, the joys of parenting are coming fast and furious, but they will fill your life with meaning and your heart with love.

Multiples after Infertility

Perhaps you've come to this point after a long battle with infertility. It's not surprising; the recent rise in the multiple birth rate is directly attributable to advances in reproductive technology. Finding yourself pregnant with two, three, or more babies after an arduous struggle just to conceive one can leave you with some conflicted feelings.

ESSENTIAL

You're not alone. It's estimated that 1 in 5 in vitro fertilization (IVF) procedures result in twins or more. Fertility drugs also produce their share of multiples, or about 1 in 10 or 20, depending on what type of drug is used. At that rate, you are quite likely to encounter other families who share your experience.

As you proceed through your pregnancy, you will likely find it very reassuring to connect with other parents in the same situation. During your battle with infertility, you may have felt that your fertile friends simply didn't understand your situation. Now that you're pregnant, you may feel similarly isolated and distanced from your infertility support community. But at the same time, you don't quite feel a common bond with parents who conceived spontaneously.

That's why it's important to establish a new support system, which includes other formerly infertile parents of multiples. Having an instant family after struggling to conceive even one child will create some interesting issues for parents, and you will find that talking about your feelings with folks who have faced the same challenges can be quite reassuring. Your local parents of multiples group is a good place to start. Or your fertility specialist may be able to put you in contact with other families.

Facing Your Feelings

A common aftereffect of infertility, especially after failed attempts to conceive, is a sensation of fear—fear that this success is fleeting, fear that you'll lose these babies that you've wanted so desperately, fear that your dream-come-true will disappear. Don't let a fear of disappointment or loss keep you from bonding with your babies. Embrace your pregnancy with a positive, optimistic attitude so that you can give your babies the best possible start in life.

FACT

While singletons conceived by assisted reproductive technology (ART) are three times more likely to be born prematurely, that trend does not hold true for multiples. The risks and complications associated with delivery were only slightly higher for ART twins than for those conceived naturally. A 2004 study showed that the risk of stillbirth or newborn death was actually lower for babies conceived with assisted reproduction.

Formerly infertile mothers often feel isolated from their peer parents when the talk turns to complaining about the negative aspects of motherhood. As someone who had to work very hard to have children, you may now feel that you don't deserve to complain about the aches and pains of pregnancy, the discomfort of labor and recovery, or the trials and tribulations of raising multiples. You asked for this, and you got it—the good and the bad. After years of desperate wishing, you can't understand how other mothers feel resentful of or frustrated by their children. You're sure you will never feel that way!

Don't judge other parents for their complaints. Deep down, they love and want their children, and they don't mean to appear insensitive or ungrateful. And don't be a martyr. Pregnancy and parenthood aren't pretty sometimes. As much as you yearned for it, you don't have to like every minute of it. Give yourself permission to join in the moaning of woeful parents, and enjoy being part of it.

Some parents feel that after working so hard to have their multiples, they can't possibly turn over their care to outsiders. Avoid that kind of "do-it-yourself" attitude. Just as you sought out assistance to help you conceive, don't be shy about seeking help once the babies are born.

Other Issues

Another factor for couples who come to a multiple pregnancy via infertility is the financial impact. Pursuing fertility assistance can be an expensive process. When successful, it is an investment that pays off in parenthood. However, the experience can leave parents deeply in debt, a problem only compounded by the expenses of raising multiples. If you find yourself in this situation, take action to address it before it becomes uncontrollable.

As time passes and your family becomes established, you will stop feeling "different." You'll exchange the rounds of fertility drugs and injections for baby Tylenol and vaccinations. When your children are old enough, be sure to share the story of their origin with them. Tell them how special they are because you wanted them so badly and worked so hard to become a family. Having multiples is a blessing unto itself, but having them after infertility is truly an amazing miracle.

Single Parents of Multiples

If you are facing multiple pregnancy and parenthood without a partner, you are likely all too aware of the additional challenges that lie ahead. You will be outnumbered, with more babies than adults in the household. You're going to need extra help, during pregnancy and beyond. It's never too early to start making arrangements for assistance. As your pregnancy progresses, a loss of mobility and a lack of energy may keep you from being productive.

Most mothers require some sort of help during labor and delivery. If the father of your babies is unable or unwilling to provide support, ask a relative or trusted friend to assume the role of labor coach. You can also hire a doula as a source of support.

However, the period of time when you will most require help is during your babies' infancy. With only two hands, it will be quite a challenge to manage the care of multiple newborns. You may want to consider live-in help for a few weeks or months. If you can afford it, hire a nanny or night nurse to provide assistance. As the months pass and you become adept at single-handedly caring for your multiples, you will likely find that your need for help decreases.

In parenting, a partner provides emotional as well as physical support. Joining a support group where you can share advice and companionship with other single parents can fill that role for you. A list of resources for single parents is included in Appendix A.

Adopting Multiples

There are many routes by which a family adopts multiples. It could be an international adoption, where you open your home to encompass needy children from another part of the world. Or maybe you became the legal parents of additional children due to circumstances that left their biological parents unable to care for them.

No matter how it came to pass, this unique and special way of forging a family has its own set of challenges and obstacles to overcome. For parents in this situation, the need for support is great. It's important to seek out resources that address the special concerns of adoptive parents, as well as those aimed at parents of multiples.

Sometimes adoptive parents perceive a lack of acceptance from fellow parents of multiples, and identify more closely with other adoptive families. Fortunately, both types of support are accessible in most locales. Your local parents of multiples organizations may include members who have adopted multiples. In addition, organizations for adoptive parents provide support throughout the adoption process. Networking with these other parents who have similar experiences can be very valuable.

FACT

There are more than 900 adoption-related support groups in North America. These groups give parents the opportunity to share their experiences and emotions, as well as information.

International Adoptions

In some cultures, the birth of twins or multiples is not a welcomed or cherished event. In societies plagued by famine or poverty, multiples may simply be too many mouths to feed. A desperate mother may abandon one or more of the babies in an attempt to provide for the other members of her family. In countries where male offspring are accorded precedence over females, there can be an abundance of discarded daughters, including sets of female twins or the female of a set of boy-girl twins. Many loving families welcome the opportunity to adopt and raise these children.

If you proceed with an international adoption of multiples, you may have some interesting cultural and linguistic issues. It can be very helpful to study the language and customs of the country of adoption. If your adopted multiples are too young to remember their birth country, you may wish to develop some special family traditions to commemorate their heritage.

Not Quite Twins

On occasion, adoption may produce a situation where two siblings are the same age, but biologically unrelated. Although not technically defined as multiples, they may be raised as such, and will come to share many of the characteristics of twins, triplets, or the like. For example, if a couple in the process of adopting an infant becomes pregnant, their biological child and their adopted child could be extremely close in age, only weeks or months apart. Or a blended family might include children and stepchildren of the same age. In situations like this, it's perfectly acceptable to treat the children as twins or multiples, assuming that they are comfortable with that role.

Multiple Multiples

A very few families are lucky enough to be blessed with multiple multiples: more than one set of twins, triplets, or more. It's hard to believe that some families could hit the jackpot more than once, but it does happen. With the increase in multiple birth mostly attributed to assisted reproduction, the trend in multiple multiples hasn't experienced the same drastic uprising. Often couples who have multiples after a complicated process of conception assistance don't go through the process more than once.

But in families that have a natural tendency toward twinning, it's not surprising. The factors that influence multiple birth—hyperovulation due to advanced maternal age, fertility drugs, or genetic predisposition—remain elevated with subsequent pregnancies. If you have an increased likelihood of conceiving twins once, your chances are good that it will happen again.

ALERT!

Experts claim that a previous twin pregnancy quadruples a woman's risk of having them again. That is, a woman who has already had twins is four times as likely to have them again as a woman who has only given birth to singletons, or has never had children at all.

However, those identified factors only apply to dizygotic (fraternal) twinning. If your existing multiples are monozygotic (identical), then your chances should be the same as anyone else's that your next pregnancy will be multiples, right?

Except that there are two aspects of having multiples to consider: your chance of conceiving multiples and your chance of sustaining a multiple pregnancy. The first of these refers to the process of multiple sperm meeting the multiple eggs, or the chance of a fertilized egg splitting. The second concerns the ability of the fertilized egg(s) to travel to the uterus, implant, and begin to develop.

Some theories hold that having a previous twin or multiple pregnancy increases the odds of having a subsequent one based on the second factor: the mother's ability to sustain the pregnancy. The reasoning is based on the high number of twin conceptions that never result in the live birth of two babies. Early ultrasound has allowed the detection of multiple embryos within a few days after conception. However, it is estimated that only 20 percent of those early pregnancies produce two or more live babies nine months later.

Because the body may consider a multiple pregnancy to be an abnormality, it may reject the pregnancy, resulting in miscarriage (a total loss of the pregnancy) or vanishing twin syndrome (reabsorption of one or more of the embryos, leaving one healthy, surviving fetus). However, if the multiple pregnancy does persevere, the body accepts it as a normal state, and subsequent twin pregnancies are more likely to thrive.

FACT

The popular children's book series *The Bobbsey Twins* featured a family with two sets of fraternal twins. Nan and Bert were about four years older than their younger twin siblings, Flossie and Freddie, when the series began, but in subsequent books their ages ranged from six to twelve.

Whether that theory holds true or not, there have been cases where families produced an incredible assortment of multiples. A Russian woman in the eighteenth century reportedly gave birth to an astonishing amount: four sets of quadruplets, seven sets of triplets, and sixteen sets of twins. Several families in the state of Pennsylvania have had twins followed by higher order multiples. Most recently, the three-year old Gosselin twins were joined by a set of sextuplets when their three brothers and three sisters were born in early 2004. In 2002 a set of quintuplets were born to a Pennsylvania family with five-year-old twin boys. Most common, however, are double sets of twins within a family. About one in three thousand women give birth to two sets of twins. Meanwhile, one in 500,000 will have three sets.

For families having multiples again, the news can be a mixed blessing. On the one hand, you are all too aware of the hardships, and with other children to care for, you may not look forward to a complicated pregnancy or the added chaos of infant multiples. Yet you've been through the experience before—you know what to expect, and many of your worries and concerns can be set aside. As an experienced parent, you've mastered the basics of baby care, and have developed efficient routines and shortcuts. You're an old pro, and can look forward to the additional joy that more multiples will bring to your unique family.

Loss of a Multiple

Unfortunately, the complications that besiege multiple pregnancies sometimes result in the loss of one or more babies. Miscarriage, stillbirth, intra-uterine fetal death, prematurity, and SIDS are all more common in multiples than in singletons. In addition, monozygotic multiples face potentially fatal complications such as twin-to-twin transfusion syndrome and conjoined twinning. No matter when the loss occurs, whether in the first trimester or after birth, it presents a complex situation for parents and any surviving multiples.

Losing a multiple is a unique kind of bereavement. The parents may not deal with the loss in the same way as parents mourning for a singleton. In addition to losing a precious child, they may also grieve the loss of the multiples' identity, as "the twins" or "the triplets." For example, when one of a set of triplets dies, the remaining two children may be classified as twins by society, but their parents will always consider them incomplete triplets.

What are the chances that not all of a group of multiples will survive?
Statistics on multiple mortality are hard to come by, but one study showed that one in twenty mothers of twins will lose one or both of the babies in the last half of her pregnancy.

Parents dealing with the loss of one or more multiples may follow an atypical pace and pattern of grief. When there are surviving multiples, they are told to focus on their living children and to consider themselves lucky that there are survivors. They'll experience a wide range of emotion, including anger toward other families with multiples or guilt about their inability to prevent their child's death. They may be extremely overprotective of their surviving child(ren) or, conversely, emotionally disconnected because the remaining multiple(s) are a constant reminder of the loss. They may try to deny the loss by focusing intently on the survivor(s). Or they may feel intensely determined to keep alive the memory of the lost babies, to the exclusion of other children.

CLIMB, the Center for Loss in Multiple Birth, recommends some strategies for parents of multiples trying to cope with the loss of one or all of their babies. First, they urge parents to take the opportunity to hold and spend time with each baby, even while dying or after death. Often in the crisis of a medical situation, parents of multiples are denied a peaceful opportunity to say goodbye to their child. This special time may take place at the hospital or later, at the funeral home. They also encourage parents to record the events of their lost child's life, no matter how brief, by taking pictures or videos, and by collecting mementos, such as a footprint, lock of hair, hospital bracelet, or blanket.

As part of the grieving process, many parents find it helpful to obtain a medical conclusion as to what went wrong. An autopsy or pregnancy loss evaluation can provide answers that alleviate the parents' sense of guilt or blame, as well as assist them in making decisions regarding future pregnancy care.

ESSENTIAL

Many parents who experience a loss find it comforting to send out a special announcement that explains the birth and death of their multiple(s). Samples of this type of correspondence can be found at CLIMB's Web site, *www.climb-support.org*.

Grief counseling is highly recommended for parents who experience the loss of a multiple. Your hospital may be able to suggest a local resource, or CLIMB can put you in touch with counselors or support groups in your area. Often, delayed feelings of grief or depression surface on significant dates, such as birthdays or anniversaries, and parents continue to need support for years after the loss.

If there are surviving multiples, you will likely be very concerned with helping these children cope with the loss of their co-twin or co-multiple. It can be a difficult parenting challenge. It's important to be honest with children about their origin in life. Even if young children don't seem to recall the presence of a twin or co-multiple, some research indicates that a subconscious awareness does exist. These children may grow up with a sense of something missing in their lives. They may experience survivor guilt, wondering why they survived when their sibling did not. The Twinless Twins International Support Group, established by a man who lost his twin brother in an accident, can provide support to children in this situation as well as to their parents.

Chapter 21

Finding Support During Pregnancy and Beyond

Having multiples is much more manageable when you take a team approach. You simply can't do it alone. Assistance comes in a variety of forms: professional services, neighbors and friends, babysitters, medical advisers, or family members. Figuring out what kind of help will be most beneficial is half the battle.

Joining a Support Group

One of the first things you should do upon discovering that you are having twins, triplets, or more is to develop a support group of families in similar circumstances. Talking to parents who have been through the experience will not only prove reassuring, but will help you prepare to face the challenges ahead. Luckily for parents of multiples, a vast network of fellow families exists throughout the world. You'll find multiples clubs and parenting organizations in nearly every region of the United States, and in most countries of the world.

These groups evolved in recognition of the tremendous benefit of sharing support and advice among fellow families of twins and other multiples. Parents of multiples face unique challenges that parents of singletons don't understand. They have much to gain from the experience of others.

FACT

The National Organization of Mothers of Twins Clubs (NOMOTC) is a nonprofit organization founded in 1960 to promote the special aspects of child development that relate specifically to multiple birth children. To find a club in your area, call the NOMOTC (877-243-2276) or stop by their Web site at *www.nomotc.org*.

The Benefits of Belonging

In the United States, the NOMOTC is a network of nearly 500 clubs, representing over 20,000 individual families. Most NOMOTC-affiliated clubs offer monthly meetings, programs about parenting multiples, resource libraries, and clothing/equipment sales. Some groups are large and busy, while others are small and casual. Other opportunities that the clubs might offer include

- Playgroups organized by community or multiples' ages
- Meal delivery for families with newborns
- Outings for moms or couples
- Babysitting co-op

- Monthly newsletter
- Family activities such as picnics or visits to theme parks
- Mentor or buddy programs for expectant mothers
- Community discount program
- Service opportunities benefiting the community or needy families
- Regional and national conferences with speakers, discussion forums, and classes about parenting multiples

Membership in a local organization gives you the additional benefit of national membership. In addition to NOMOTC affiliates, there are numerous independent clubs. If you are having difficulty locating a club in your area, inquire through your physician or hospital; they can usually put you in touch with someone.

Usually, families that are expecting multiples or have newborns are invited to visit a monthly meeting without obligation. If you decide to join, there is usually a membership fee to become a member and take advantage of the club's benefits. Part of the fee will be designated for the national and regional club, while the remainder is used to fund the local club's activities.

QUESTION?

I'm not really a "joiner." Will I still find a club useful?
Even if you don't like to commit to committees, it's worth investigating the multiples organization in your area. You can usually visit a meeting or talk by phone with a club representative before making a commitment. These organizations exist to serve parents, not obligate them, so don't worry that you'll be expected to participate in anything you're uncomfortable with.

Who Belongs?

Club designations vary. Some are called "parents of multiples clubs" while others specify "mothers of twins." In reality, the majority of programming and support is generally aimed at the mother, although some clubs include grandparents, adopted parents, and caregivers of multiples.

Some larger cities have a designated group for families with triplets, quadruplets, or higher order multiples. If your area does not offer such a group, two national organizations may offer some support. The Triplet Connection offers information packets and presents an annual conference. Membership in MOST (Mothers of Supertwins) entitles you to receive phone support, access to online resources, and a quarterly magazine.

Seeking Support Online

The Internet has opened up a whole new world for parents of multiples. Up-to-date information is readily available from the comfort of your living room at any time of the day or night. In addition, you can enjoy immediate access to fellow parents from around the world without worrying about jet lag or even whether you've had time to shower that day.

Although books like this one are invaluable collections of resources and facts, the Internet has the added benefit of providing up-to-the-minute updates about multiple birth issues, including crucial medical advances. If you encounter a specific problem in your pregnancy, such as twin-to-twin transfusion syndrome, or are fighting the battle against preterm labor, you can research in-depth explanations about possible treatments and options.

ALERT!

Be sure to discuss any medical information you find on the Internet with your doctor. Just because something is published online doesn't ensure that it is accurate, or appropriate, for your individual circumstances.

In addition to factual information, the Internet is a tremendous human resource. You've already learned that fellow parents are your best source of advice, and the Internet puts that font of wisdom literally at your fingertips. You can connect with other parents via chats, discussion forums, message boards, e-mail, and instant messaging. You can communicate as part of a group or one-on-one with individuals.

The Welcoming Web

So how do you find fellow parents online? Start at Web sites focused on the topic of parenting multiples; many have community features that connect users via chats or message boards. Chats are scheduled events, bringing together individual users at a designated time in an online chat room where they can participate in real-time interactive discussions. Message boards—also called discussion boards or forums—are ongoing discussions where users add their comments and responses in the form of posts.

FACT

Look for venues that are moderated to keep things clean. In addition, choose forums with plenty of recent responses so that you know someone is paying attention and there is enough traffic to sustain conversation.

Online mailing lists about multiple birth allow families to communicate via e-mail. Some lists take the form of informational newsletters, while others are more interactive in nature. If you have inquiries about a specific topic or desire the ability to respond to comments, you'll want to subscribe to the latter.

Online communication has many benefits for families with multiples. First, it's available when you are, twenty-four hours a day and seven days a week. When you have newborn twins, triplets, or more in the house, you can't keep banker's hours. You may be asleep from nine A.M. until noon, and wide awake at three A.M. Using e-mail or other online communication tools allows you to keep in touch with people according to your schedule. If you find a few free minutes while the babies nap, you can go online and accomplish several tasks that would take hours to do offline: share photos, pay bills, shop, find a recipe for dinner, get information on baby care, network with other parents, send out e-mail updates about the babies' progress, and more!

Several online resources are included in Appendix A. Spend some time browsing to discover a world of information about twins and multiples, including medical resources, parenting advice, multiple-themed merchandise, online communities, and much more. A word of caution is in order, however. Just as in the "real" world, the virtual world has its share of hazards. Be wary of people you encounter online. Identity falsification is rampant; it's difficult to confirm that the person on your computer screen is who they claim to be. Use common sense: don't send money to, agree to meet with, or become emotionally invested in anyone you meet online without checking out their credentials.

Prenatal and Childbirth Classes

One of the most stereotypical traditions of pregnancy is attending a childbirth class with your partner. You lie on pillows on the floor, practice funny breathing, and dreamily anticipate the joy of welcoming your new baby. Unfortunately, the reality of these classes is that they are not always relevant to the multiple birth experience. Preterm labor or bed rest may prohibit you from making it to a class if you wait until the third trimester. A scheduled c-section would eliminate the need for labor management instruction. However, childbirth preparation classes aren't entirely a waste of time for parents of multiples. There are several ways that you can derive benefit from formal instruction.

What to Expect

First-time parents are usually the most common candidates for childbirth education. If your multiples will be your first born—as well as second, and maybe third—then you should definitely consider a class that covers the basics of labor and delivery. Some of the things that might be covered are

- Different methods of labor management, such as Bradley or Lamaze
- Explanation of the stages of labor
- Anesthesia and medication
- Complications
- Relaxation and pain management

Some classes also address the mother's postpartum care, newborn care, cesarean birth procedures, or the father's role. If you've experienced a previous pregnancy and normal delivery, you may find that this type of beginner class is redundant. You may be more interested in a refresher class, VBAC (vaginal birth after cesarean) preparation, sibling adjustment training, or other programs for veteran parents.

You may find it helpful to team up with one or two other couples who are also having twins or more and enroll in a class together. That way, you're not the exception in the class. Don't be afraid to inform the instructor about your multiple pregnancy, and inquire as to how each topic relates to a multiple birth.

Information about childbirth education is usually available from your doctor or hospital. It can be helpful to take a class at the hospital where you plan to deliver the babies because policies and procedures often vary from one location to the next. You may also have the opportunity to tour your hospital's maternity and nursery departments so that you are familiar with the facilities.

Most singleton families wait until the third trimester to enroll in birthing classes, but parents of multiples are advised not to put it off! If you are expecting twins, you should plan to complete your class before the end of your second trimester. If you are expecting triplets or more, the end of the first trimester is not too early to begin your training. Preterm labor or bed rest restrictions may preclude you from attending later in the pregnancy.

Multiple-Specific Classes

In recent years, as the number of multiple births has increased, greater attention has been focused on the unique circumstances of parents of multiples. Fortunately, that has resulted in more opportunities for multiple-birth families to receive education specific to their situation. Classes on managing multiple pregnancy, labor and delivery with multiples, and newborn care of multiples are becoming more readily available.

Marvelous Multiples is a national network of classes designed for parents of multiples. Classes are available in most states in the United States as well as throughout Canada. Going beyond childbirth education, it covers many vital topics about multiples including

- Physical and emotional challenges of multiple pregnancy
- Variances in labor, delivery, and recovery with multiples
- Newborn care of multiples
- Networking with other families

Some programs are sponsored by a nonprofit organization and are available for free. Others charge a fee. Some of the costs may be offset by your insurance coverage. Many of the programs are associated with hospitals or local mothers of multiples clubs, either of which can provide full details regarding class schedules and registration. You can also check Marvelous Multiples' Web site (*www.marvelousmultiples.com*) for class locations.

FACT

Marvelous Multiples recommends that mothers attend a class before their twenty-second week of pregnancy, in order to gain the maximum benefit from the information. Classes usually cover about eight hours of material and can be presented in eight-week, four-week, or weekend sessions. Usually a discussion panel led by experienced twin or higher order multiple parents concludes the class.

Help from Family and Friends

Many families with multiples are fortunate to find themselves the beneficiaries of numerous offers of assistance from friends and relatives. Some even have the support of an entire neighborhood or church community. However, just because help is available doesn't mean that it is helpful. You'll want to be sure that you accept help in ways that make life with multiples easier, not more complicated.

Help During Pregnancy

There are many instances throughout a multiple pregnancy when you can use a bit of assistance. Because mothers of multiples experience more complications, they may find themselves restricted to bed or hospitalized at some point during their pregnancy. To a lesser extreme, they may simply find that their physical symptoms are intensified to the point where normal activities become uncomfortable and everyday chores and responsibilities may become a burden. During those times, it's very helpful to have some assistance lined up, such as meal preparation, errand running, or child care for older siblings.

It can also be a very emotional time, with lots of anxiety about what lies ahead. Pregnancy is a good time to call upon friends for reassurance and encouragement. See a funny movie or laugh about old times together. A mother's emotional state has a great deal of influence over her physical condition; friends can play an important role in keeping her spirits uplifted.

Help after the Babies Come Home

Once your babies arrive and your family's focus shifts to round-the-clock newborn nurturing, opportunities abound for outside assistance. Don't be afraid to accept help, and don't hesitate to ask for it, either. People genuinely want to help, and you genuinely need it. Take everyone up on their offers, but utilize the help in such a way that it serves your needs.

ALERT!

No matter what kind of help you have, don't underestimate the need to protect the babies from harmful germs. Tiny newborns, especially if they were preterm, are particularly susceptible to dangerous infections due to underdeveloped immunity. Explain proper hand-washing techniques to your helpers, and enforce a policy that requires them to wash up before touching the babies.

First, be specific about what you need. Nearly everyone wants to "help" by holding or rocking a baby. Sometimes that's nice if it offers you a break to accomplish something else, but be realistic about how helpful it really is. Do you need help finishing chores? Or caring for other children? Some families with higher order multiples may require help around the clock, just to get all the babies fed and changed!

Some other forms of assistance you might want to consider are

- Extra hands at feeding times
- Telephone answering and filtering calls
- Photography (taking, developing, and/or uploading pictures to the Web)
- Meals for the family
- Laundry
- Yard work
- Errand running (grocery shopping, post office, dry cleaner)
- Transportation (to doctor visits for you, or to school and activities for older children)
- Bath-time assistance
- Care for other siblings (homework help, playtime)

Once you have established your needs, organize your helpers. Preferably have someone else organize the help. The less you have to worry about anything other than the babies, the better. An efficient organizer is the best helper you can have. Have her create a list of your needs, then match helpers according to their abilities and availabilities.

Helpers will appreciate having a specified opportunity to help. For example, saying, "Please come by at 7 P.M. on Thursday to help feed the babies and put them to bed" lets your friends know exactly what is expected of them. It allows you to receive help at the times you need it most, while discouraging unwelcome drop-in visitors when you're sleeping or otherwise occupied.

Try to determine ahead of time when you will need the most assistance. Most families find that they require the majority of help in the first few weeks after their babies are born and/or when they bring them home. Fortunately, that's usually when the most offers for help are made. After a few months, the need for help diminishes somewhat as the family adjusts and establishes a routine. However, you may find that you would appreciate some form of ongoing or occasional assistance for several months longer, perhaps a weekly meal delivery, occasional babysitting so that Mom and Dad can enjoy a night out (or in!), or transportation to the babies' three-month checkup with the pediatrician.

But I Don't Want Help!

If you are very independent—or organized—you may not wish to have your home and private family life invaded by outsiders. That's okay, too. Don't refuse all offers of help outright, however. Instead, specify ways that meet your needs while respecting your privacy and comfort level. Perhaps you would find it helpful to have a friend pick up some items at the grocery store rather than prepare a meal. Or maybe you'd rather that your mother-in-law help care for your older children rather than the new babies. Make a mental note of the friends and family members who offer their help so that you can call on them down the road if you do find yourself in need at a later time.

Professional Services and Counseling

Sometimes volunteer help simply isn't enough. There are times when you'll need to call in a professional. If you can afford to pay for help, you may find it well worth the cost. Decide how your money will be best spent by considering what services you can turn over to another party while you concentrate on the activities that mean the most to you.

FACT

Ongoing or occasional cleaning assistance makes a great gift for new parents. If you're making up a wish list, go ahead and include it! Because of the cost, a group of gift-givers may wish to combine their resources and present the gift together.

Help Around the House

When multiples join a household, things change forever. If you've been accustomed to cleaning and maintaining your home, you may find that your time to devote to it is severely diminished once your babies arrive. While housework still needs to be done, it is one of the responsibilities that most people don't mind giving up. Paying for a cleaning service to maintain your home removes the burden and lets you focus your attention on your new babies. Even if you don't need ongoing service, a one-time thorough cleaning would help you put your home in order and get your expanded family off to a good start.

In addition to housekeeping, there are several other home responsibilities that can be turned over to professionals in order to free up expectant or new parents' time. For example, meal preparation services are becoming very popular options for busy families. Professional landscapers can take over yard work duties. Pet sitters can relieve you of pet chores such as feeding, walking, and cleaning up. Professional organizers can help you streamline your routines and reduce clutter in your home to make your lifestyle more efficient.

Help with the Babies

Professional advice and assistance with caring for your newborn multiples can literally be a lifesaver. First-time parents, parents of premature multiples, or parents of infants with special medical needs will greatly benefit from the personal attention of a hired nurse or caregiver, such as a doula.

Doulas provide a comforting, supportive presence to mothers—and fathers—during childbirth, but are also available for postpartum care. As an objective and neutral party, they act as an advocate for the family and an intermediary between the parents and the medical staff. Postpartum doulas assist the mother with breastfeeding, recuperation from delivery, and newborn care. Most postpartum doulas charge by the hour, so you have the option of procuring as little or as much service as you require. Even a one-hour visit with a postpartum doula can boost new parents' confidence and provide valuable information about caring for their newborns. A short-term investment in professional help may assist you in becoming better parents in the long run.

With sleep deprivation an issue for so many new parents of multiples, the promise of a good night's sleep may be worth the cost of hiring a night nurse—a professional nurse who will come to your home to care for the babies throughout the nighttime hours so you and your partner can sleep. Costs vary, but even one night of uninterrupted sleep can improve parents' perspective and equip them to cope with their babies going forward.

Few families require around-the-clock care, but many find it useful to have an occasional visit from a postpartum doula or nurse. Your insurance may help cover the costs of these services, so be sure to investigate your options before ruling it out.

Counseling Services

Finally, don't overlook your mental health as you adjust to your newly expanded family. Having twins or multiples can be extremely stressful. It may prove tremendously helpful to find someone to talk to about your feelings. For some individuals, talking to a friend, relative, or fellow parent may be sufficient. Others, however, may require psychological support from a professional. Families who experience any of the following would be good candidates for professional counseling:

- Complicated pregnancy with high levels of stress or anxiety
- Loss of a twin or multiple
- Preterm labor resulting in premature or ill babies
- Selective reduction
- Postpartum depression
- Trouble adjusting to the demands of caring for multiple babies
- Marital problems

Serious consequences, including depression or divorce, can result if you let your emotional issues remain unresolved. Parents often neglect their own needs in their efforts to care for their children, but receiving support from a counselor or psychologist can only enhance your parenting. Your doctor or your local multiples club can steer you toward professionals who have experience helping new parents and families with multiples.

Appendix A

Recommended Resources

Additional Reading

Agnew, Connie L., Klein, Alan H., and Ganon, Jill Alison. *Twins! Pregnancy, Birth and the First Year of Life* (HarperCollins, 1997)

Bowers, Nancy. *The Multiple Pregnancy Sourcebook* (Contemporary Books, 2001)

Ford-Martin, Paula. *The Everything® Pregnancy Book, 2nd Edition* (Adams Media, 2003)

Gromada, Karen Kerkhoff. *Mothering Multiples: Breastfeeding and Caring for Twins or More* (La Leche League International, 1999)

Kohl, Susan. *Twin Stories: Their Mysterious and Unique Bond* (Wildcat Canyon Press, 2001)

Laut, William and Laut, Sheila. *Raising Multiple Birth Children* (Chandler House Press, 1999)

Leiter, Gila. *Everything You Need to Know to Have a Healthy Twin Pregnancy* (Dell Publishing, 2000)

Luke, Barbara. *Every Pregnant Woman's Guide to Preventing Preterm Labor* (Author's Choice Press, 2002)

Luke, Barbara and Eberlein, Tamara. *When You're Expecting Twins, Triplets or More* (Perennial, 2004)

Lyons, Elizabeth. *Ready or Not, Here We Come! The Real Experts' Cannot-Live-Without Guide to the First Year with Twins* (Finn-Phyllis Press, 2003)

Malmstrom, Pamela Maxwell and Poland, Janet. *The Art of Parenting Twins: The Unique Joys and Challenges of Raising Twins and Other Multiples* (Ballantine Books, 1999)

Moskwinski, Rebecca E. (Ed.) *Twins to Quints: The Complete Manual for Parents of Multiple Birth Children* (Harpeth House Publishing, 2002)

Noble, Elizabeth. *Having Twins and More* (Houghton Mifflin, 2003)

Novotny, Pamela Patrick. *The Joy of Twins and Other Multiple Births* (Crown Publishers, 1994)

Pearlman, Eileen M. and Ganon, Jill Alison. *Raising Twins from Birth Through Adolescence: What Parents Want to Know (and What Twins Want to Tell Them)* (HarperResource, 2000)

Segal, Nancy A. *Entwined Lives* (Plume, 2000)

Sipes, Nancy J. and Sipes, Janna S. *Dancing Naked in Front of the Fridge and Other Lessons from Twins* (FairWinds Press, 1998)

Tinglof, Christina Baglivi. *Double Duty: The Parents' Guide to Raising Twins from Pregnancy Through the School Years* (Contemporary Books, 1998)

Tracy, Amy E. *The Pregnancy Bed Rest Book* (Berkeley Publishing Group, 2001)

Twins Magazine
(Published six times a year.)
(888) 55-TWINS or (303) 290-8500
twins.customer.service@businessword.com
www.twinsmagazine.com

Online Resources

Bed Rest

Sidelines Pregnancy Support
P.O. Box 1808
Laguna Beach, CA 92652
(888) 447-4754 or (949) 497-5598
sidelines@sidelines.org
www.sidelines.org

Breastfeeding Support

International Lactation Consultant Association
1500 Sunday Drive
Suite 102
Raleigh, NC 27607
(919) 787-5181
info@ilca.org
www.ilca.org

La Leche League International
1400 N. Meacham Road
Schamburg, IL 60173-4808
(847) 519-7730 or (800) LALECHE
www.lalecheleague.org

Medela, Inc.
1101 Corporate Drive
McHenry, IL 60050
(800) 435-8316 or (815) 363-1166
customer.service@medela.com
www.medela.com

Childbirth Education and Support

Doulas of North America (DONA)
P.O. Box 626
Jasper, IN 47547
(888) 788-DONA
referrals@dona.org
www.dona.org

Marvelous Multiples
Nancy Bowers, RN
P.O. Box 381164
Birmingham, AL 35238
(205) 437-3575
marvmult@aol.com
www.marvelousmultiples.com

Clubs for Parents of Multiples

National Organization of Mothers of Twins Clubs (NOMOTC)
P.O. Box 438
Thompson Station, TN 37179-0438
(877) 243-2276
info@nomotc.org
www.nomotc.org

Multiple Births Canada
P.O. Box 432
Wasaga Beach, Ontario
Canada L0L 2P0
(705) 429-0901
office@multiplebirthscanada.org
www.multiplebirthscanada.org

Conjoined Twins

Conjoined Twins International
Will L. Degeraty
P.O. Box 10895
Prescott, AZ 86304-0895
(928) 445-2777
dwdegeraty@myexcel.com
www.conjoinedtwinsint.com

General Information on Multiples

Guide to Parenting Multiples at About.com
multiples.guide@about.com
multiples.about.com

Twinstuff.com
www.twinstuff.com

TwinsWorld
www.twinsworld.com

Multiple Birth: Prenatal Education and Bereavement Support
www.multiplebirthsfamilies.com

Twins-L Listserve
www.twinslist.org

Higher Order Multiples

Mothers of Supertwins (MOST)
P.O. Box 951
Brentwood, NY 11717
(631) 859-1110
info@MOSTonline.org
www.mostonline.org

Triplet Connection
Janet Bleyl, President
P.O. Box 693392
Stockton, CA 95269-3392
(209) 474-0885
janet@tripletconnection.org
www.tripletconnection.org

Loss of a Multiple

Center for Loss in Multiple Birth (CLIMB)
Jean Kollantai
P.O. Box 91377
Anchorage AK 99509
(907) 222-5321
climb@pobox.alaska.net
www.climb-support.org

Twinless Twins International Support Group
P.O. Box 980481
Ypsilanti, MI 48198-0481
(888) 205-8962
contact@twinlesstwins.org
www.twinlesstwins.org

Monoamniotic Twins

Monoamniotic.org
momo@monoamniotic.org
www.monoamniotic.org

Prematurity

American Association for Premature Infants (AAPI)
P.O. Box 46371
Cincinnati, OH 45241
(513) 956-4331

The Alexis Foundation
P.O. Box 1126
Birmingham, MI 48012-1126
(248) 543-4169 or (877) ALEXIS-0
thealexisfoundation@prodigy.net
✍*pages.prodigy.net/thealexisfoundation/
THEALEXIS1.html*

PreemieParents.com
✍*www.preemieparents.com*

PreemieTwins.com
✍*www.preemietwins.com*

Products for Twins and Multiples

**By-My-Side Safety Harness
for Twins by TommiGuard**
tommiguard@yahoo.com
✍*www.tommiguard.com*

Double Decker Stroller, Inc.
(239) 543-1582
info@doubledeckerstroller.com
✍*www.doubledeckerstroller.com*

Double Blessings
(800) 584-TWIN or (619) 441-1873
info@doubleblessings.com
✍*www.doubleblessings.com*

Great Baby Products
(425) 427-5600
twins@greatbabyproducts.com
✍*www.greatbabyproducts.com*

Multiple Trends
(800) 567-9559
info@multipletrends.com
✍*www.multipletrends.com*

More Than One, Inc.
(800) 388-8946
morthn1@aol.com
✍*www.morethan1.com*

Baby Trilogy, Inc.
(888) 874-9596
customerservice@cornercrib.com
✍*www.babytrilogy.com*

RunAbout Strollers
(435) 462-7466
jableyl@tripletconnection.org
✍*www.tripletconnection.org/st_runab.html*

Research and Support Organizations

Center for Study of Multiple Birth
Dr. Louis G. Keith
Suite 464, 333 E. Superior Street
Chicago, IL 60611
(312) 926-7498
lgk396@northwestern.edu
✍*www.multiplebirth.com*

International Twins Association
Lynn Long and Lori Stewart
6898 Channel Road N.E.
Minneapolis, MN 55432
(612) 571-3022
ITAConvention@aol.com
✍*www.intltwins.org*

California Twin Study
Thomas Mack, MD, MPH
USC/Norris Comprehensive
Cancer Center
1441 Eastlake Avenue, MS 44
Los Angeles, CA 90033-0800
🖱http://twins.usc.edu

International Society for Twin Studies
The Louisville Twins Study
Health Sciences Center
University of Louisville
P.O. Box 35260
Louisville, KY 40294
apmath01@ulkyvm.louisville.edu

Mid-Atlantic Twin Registry
Virginia Commonwealth University
P.O. Box 980003
Richmond, VA 23298-0003
(800) URA-TWIN
twinreg@hsc.vcu.edu
🖱www.matr.gen.vcu.edu

University of Minnesota Twin Study
Dr. Thomas J. Bouchard, Jr.
Twins-Reared-Apart Project
University of Minnesota
Minneapolis, MN 55455
bouch001@maroon.tc.umn.edu

Wisconsin Twin Project
Kathryn S. Lemery
Waisman Center
1500 Highland Avenue
University of Wisconsin-Madison
Madison, WI 53705
(608) 265-2674

wisconsintwins@waisman.wisc.edu
🖱psych.wisc.edu/wtp/

The Twins Foundation
P.O. Box 6043
Providence, RI 02940-6043
(401) 751-TWIN [(401) 751-8946]
twins@twinsfoundation.com
🖱www.twinsfoundation.com

Twin Services Consulting
P.O. Box 10066
Berkeley, CA 94709
(510) 524-0863
twinservices@juno.com
🖱www.twinservices.org

Twinsight
1137 Second Street
Suite 109
Santa Monica, CA 90403
(310) 458-1373
epearlman@twinsight.com
🖱www.twinsight.com

Single Parents

Single Parenting Guide at About.com
singleparents.guide@about.com
🖱singleparents.about.com

Parents Without Partners
1650 South Dixie Highway, Suite 510
Boca Raton, FL 33432
(561) 391-8833
pwp@jti.net
🖱www.parentswithoutpartners.org

Twin-to-Twin Transfusion Syndrome

The Twin-to-Twin Transfusion Syndrome Foundation
411 Longbeach Parkway
Bay Village, OH 44140
(800) 815-9211 or (440) 899-8887
diagnosed@tttsfoundation.org
www.tttsfoundation.org

Florida Perinatal Associates Fetal Therapy Program
Dr. Ruben Quintero
13601 Bruce B. Downs Boulevard
Suite 250
Tampa, FL 33613
(888) 338-2577 or (813) 872-3982
quintero@fetalmd.com
www.fetalmd.com

The International Institute for the Treatment of Twin to Twin Transfusion Syndrome
Dr. Julian E. De Lia
St. Joseph Regional Medical Center
5000 West Chambers Street
Milwaukee, WI 53210-1688
www.covhealth.org

Zygosity Testing

Pro-DNA Diagnostic
(514) 253-9998 or (877) 236-6444
info@proadn.com
www.proadn.com

Affiliated Genetics, Inc.
P.O. Box 58535
Salt Lake City, UT 84158
(800) 362-5559 or (801) 582-4200
service@affiliatedgenetics.com
www.affiliatedgenetics.com

Proactive Genetics, Inc.
158R Front Street
Marblehead, MA 01945
(781) 639-5126
info@proactivegenetics.com
www.proactivegenetics.com/ zygosity.dna

Appendix B

Keeping Track: Charting Your Newborns' Progress

Use this chart to help you keep track of your babies' feedings, diaper activity, and administration of any medications each day. This form will accommodate up to four babies; print out two per day if you have quintuplets or higher.

Filling Out Your Progress Chart

At the top of each column, note the babies' names. Each time you feed and change the babies, note the time in the left-hand column. Under each baby's name, fill in the four squares.

- **Feed:** Indicate the amount of formula in ounces, or the amount of time spent breastfeeding in minutes. If breastfeeding, you may also wish to indicate which breast the baby nursed from, with an "R" to designate the right side and an "L" for the left side.
- **Med:** If any of your babies require medications, you can use this space to keep track of the dosages. Check the box when you have administered medication to make sure that each baby is getting the right dose at the right time.
- **WD:** Use this space to record the number of wet diapers since the last feeding. It's important that each baby is urinating enough to soak a diaper. A lack of wet diapers could indicate dehydration.
- **BM:** This section also represents your baby's diaper achievements. Use it to record bowel movements. You can use a tally system or just check the box after you've changed a soiled diaper.

Today's Date _____

Time	Baby A:		Baby B:		Baby C:		Baby D:	
Time	Feed:	Med:	Feed:	Med:	Feed:	Med:	Feed:	Med:
	WD:	BM:	WD:	BM:	WD:	BM:	WD:	BM:
Time	Feed:	Med:	Feed:	Med:	Feed:	Med:	Feed:	Med:
	WD:	BM:	WD:	BM:	WD:	BM:	WD:	BM:
Time	Feed:	Med:	Feed:	Med:	Feed:	Med:	Feed:	Med:
	WD:	BM:	WD:	BM:	WD:	BM:	WD:	BM:
Time	Feed:	Med:	Feed:	Med:	Feed:	Med:	Feed:	Med:
	WD:	BM:	WD:	BM:	WD:	BM:	WD:	BM:
Time	Feed:	Med:	Feed:	Med:	Feed:	Med:	Feed:	Med:
	WD:	BM:	WD:	BM:	WD:	BM:	WD:	BM:
Time	Feed:	Med:	Feed:	Med:	Feed:	Med:	Feed:	Med:
	WD:	BM:	WD:	BM:	WD:	BM:	WD:	BM:
Time	Feed:	Med:	Feed:	Med:	Feed:	Med:	Feed:	Med:
	WD:	BM:	WD:	BM:	WD:	BM:	WD:	BM:
Time	Feed:	Med:	Feed:	Med:	Feed:	Med:	Feed:	Med:
	WD:	BM:	WD:	BM:	WD:	BM:	WD:	BM:
Time	Feed:	Med:	Feed:	Med:	Feed:	Med:	Feed:	Med:
	WD:	BM:	WD:	BM:	WD:	BM:	WD:	BM:
Time	Feed:	Med:	Feed:	Med:	Feed:	Med:	Feed:	Med:
	WD:	BM:	WD:	BM:	WD:	BM:	WD:	BM:
Time	Feed:	Med:	Feed:	Med:	Feed:	Med:	Feed:	Med:
	WD:	BM:	WD:	BM:	WD:	BM:	WD:	BM:
Time	Feed:	Med:	Feed:	Med:	Feed:	Med:	Feed:	Med:
	WD:	BM:	WD:	BM:	WD:	BM:	WD:	BM:
Time	Feed:	Med:	Feed:	Med:	Feed:	Med:	Feed:	Med:
	WD:	BM:	WD:	BM:	WD:	BM:	WD:	BM:
Time	Feed:	Med:	Feed:	Med:	Feed:	Med:	Feed:	Med:
	WD:	BM:	WD:	BM:	WD:	BM:	WD:	BM:
Time	Feed:	Med:	Feed:	Med:	Feed:	Med:	Feed:	Med:
	WD:	BM:	WD:	BM:	WD:	BM:	WD:	BM:

THE EVERYTHING SERIES!

BUSINESS & PERSONAL FINANCE

Everything® Budgeting Book
Everything® Business Planning Book
Everything® Coaching and Mentoring Book
Everything® Fundraising Book
Everything® Get Out of Debt Book
Everything® Grant Writing Book
Everything® Homebuying Book, 2nd Ed.
Everything® Homeselling Book
Everything® Home-Based Business Book
Everything® Investing Book
Everything® Landlording Book
Everything® Leadership Book
Everything® Managing People Book
Everything® Negotiating Book
Everything® Online Business Book
Everything® Personal Finance Book
Everything® Personal Finance in Your 20s
    and 30s Book
Everything® Project Management Book
Everything® Real Estate Investing Book
Everything® Robert's Rules Book, $7.95
Everything® Selling Book
Everything® Start Your Own Business Book
Everything® Wills & Estate Planning Book

COOKING

Everything® Barbecue Cookbook
Everything® Bartender's Book, $9.95
Everything® Chinese Cookbook
Everything® College Cookbook
Everything® Cookbook
Everything® Diabetes Cookbook
Everything® Easy Gourmet Cookbook
Everything® Fondue Cookbook
Everything® Grilling Cookbook
Everything® Healthy Meals in Minutes
    Cookbook
Everything® Holiday Cookbook

Everything® Indian Cookbook
Everything® Low-Carb Cookbook
Everything® Low-Fat High-Flavor Cookbook
Everything® Low-Salt Cookbook
Everything® Meals for a Month Cookbook
Everything® Mediterranean Cookbook
Everything® Mexican Cookbook
Everything® One-Pot Cookbook
Everything® Pasta Cookbook
Everything® Quick Meals Cookbook
Everything® Slow Cooker Cookbook
Everything® Soup Cookbook
Everything® Thai Cookbook
Everything® Vegetarian Cookbook
Everything® Wine Book

HEALTH

Everything® Alzheimer's Book
Everything® Diabetes Book
Everything® Hypnosis Book
Everything® Low Cholesterol Book
Everything® Massage Book
Everything® Menopause Book
Everything® Nutrition Book
Everything® Reflexology Book
Everything® Stress Management Book

HISTORY

Everything® American Government Book
Everything® American History Book
Everything® Civil War Book
Everything® Irish History & Heritage Book
Everything® Middle East Book

HOBBIES & GAMES

Everything® Blackjack Strategy Book
Everything® Brain Strain Book, $9.95
Everything® Bridge Book
Everything® Candlemaking Book

Everything® Card Games Book
Everything® Cartooning Book
Everything® Casino Gambling Book, 2nd Ed.
Everything® Chess Basics Book
Everything® Crossword and Puzzle Book
Everything® Crossword Challenge Book
Everything® Cryptograms Book, $9.95
Everything® Digital Photography Book
Everything® Drawing Book
Everything® Easy Crosswords Book
Everything® Family Tree Book
Everything® Games Book, 2nd Ed.
Everything® Knitting Book
Everything® Knots Book
Everything® Motorcycle Book
Everything® Online Genealogy Book
Everything® Photography Book
Everything® Poker Strategy Book
Everything® Pool & Billiards Book
Everything® Quilting Book
Everything® Scrapbooking Book
Everything® Sewing Book
Everything® Woodworking Book
Everything® Word Games Challenge Book

HOME IMPROVEMENT

Everything® Feng Shui Book
Everything® Feng Shui Decluttering Book,
    $9.95
Everything® Fix-It Book
Everything® Homebuilding Book
Everything® Lawn Care Book
Everything® Organize Your Home Book

EVERYTHING® KIDS' BOOKS

All titles are $6.95
Everything® Kids' Animal Puzzle & Activity
    Book
Everything® Kids' Baseball Book, 3rd Ed.

All Everything® books are priced at $12.95 or $14.95, unless otherwise stated. Prices subject to change without notice.

Everything® Kids' Bible Trivia Book
Everything® Kids' Bugs Book
Everything® Kids' Christmas Puzzle
   & Activity Book
Everything® Kids' Cookbook
Everything® Kids' Halloween Puzzle
   & Activity Book
Everything® Kids' Hidden Pictures Book
Everything® Kids' Joke Book
Everything® Kids' Knock Knock Book
Everything® Kids' Math Puzzles Book
Everything® Kids' Mazes Book
Everything® Kids' Money Book
Everything® Kids' Monsters Book
Everything® Kids' Nature Book
Everything® Kids' Puzzle Book
Everything® Kids' Riddles & Brain Teasers Book
Everything® Kids' Science Experiments Book
Everything® Kids' Sharks Book
Everything® Kids' Soccer Book
Everything® Kids' Travel Activity Book

KIDS' STORY BOOKS

Everything® Bedtime Story Book
Everything® Fairy Tales Book

LANGUAGE

Everything® Conversational Japanese Book
   (with CD), $19.95
Everything® French Phrase Book, $9.95
Everything® French Verb Book, $9.95
Everything® Inglés Book
Everything® Learning French Book
Everything® Learning German Book
Everything® Learning Italian Book
Everything® Learning Latin Book
Everything® Learning Spanish Book
Everything® Sign Language Book
Everything® Spanish Grammar Book
Everything® Spanish Phrase Book, $9.95
Everything® Spanish Verb Book, $9.95

MUSIC

Everything® Drums Book (with CD), $19.95
Everything® Guitar Book
Everything® Home Recording Book
Everything® Playing Piano and Keyboards
   Book

Everything® Reading Music Book (with CD),
   $19.95
Everything® Rock & Blues Guitar Book
   (with CD), $19.95
Everything® Songwriting Book

NEW AGE

Everything® Astrology Book
Everything® Dreams Book, 2nd Ed.
Everything® Ghost Book
Everything® Love Signs Book, $9.95
Everything® Numerology Book
Everything® Paganism Book
Everything® Palmistry Book
Everything® Psychic Book
Everything® Reiki Book
Everything® Spells & Charms Book
Everything® Tarot Book
Everything® Wicca and Witchcraft Book

PARENTING

Everything® Baby Names Book
Everything® Baby Shower Book
Everything® Baby's First Food Book
Everything® Baby's First Year Book
Everything® Birthing Book
Everything® Breastfeeding Book
Everything® Father-to-Be Book
Everything® Father's First Year Book
Everything® Get Ready for Baby Book
Everything® Getting Pregnant Book
Everything® Homeschooling Book
Everything® Parent's Guide to Children
   with ADD/ADHD
Everything® Parent's Guide to Children
   with Asperger's Syndrome
Everything® Parent's Guide to Children
   with Autism
Everything® Parent's Guide to Children
   with Dyslexia
Everything® Parent's Guide to Positive
   Discipline
Everything® Parent's Guide to Raising a
   Successful Child
Everything® Parent's Guide to Tantrums
Everything® Parent's Guide to the Overweight
   Child
Everything® Parenting a Teenager Book
Everything® Potty Training Book, $9.95

Everything® Pregnancy Book, 2nd Ed.
Everything® Pregnancy Fitness Book
Everything® Pregnancy Nutrition Book
Everything® Pregnancy Organizer, $15.00
Everything® Toddler Book
Everything® Tween Book
Everything® Twins, Triplets, and More Book

PETS

Everything® Cat Book
Everything® Dachshund Book, $12.95
Everything® Dog Book
Everything® Dog Health Book
Everything® Dog Training and Tricks Book
Everything® Golden Retriever Book, $12.95
Everything® Horse Book
Everything® Labrador Retriever Book, $12.95
Everything® Poodle Book, $12.95
Everything® Pug Book, $12.95
Everything® Puppy Book
Everything® Rottweiler Book, $12.95
Everything® Tropical Fish Book

REFERENCE

Everything® Car Care Book
Everything® Classical Mythology Book
Everything® Computer Book
Everything® Divorce Book
Everything® Einstein Book
Everything® Etiquette Book
Everything® Mafia Book
Everything® Philosophy Book
Everything® Psychology Book
Everything® Shakespeare Book

RELIGION

Everything® Angels Book
Everything® Bible Book
Everything® Buddhism Book
Everything® Catholicism Book
Everything® Christianity Book
Everything® Jewish History & Heritage Book
Everything® Judaism Book
Everything® Koran Book
Everything® Prayer Book
Everything® Saints Book
Everything® Torah Book
Everything® Understanding Islam Book

All Everything® books are priced at $12.95 or $14.95, unless otherwise stated. Prices subject to change without notice.

Everything® World's Religions Book
Everything® Zen Book

SCHOOL & CAREERS

Everything® Alternative Careers Book
Everything® College Survival Book, 2nd Ed.
Everything® Cover Letter Book, 2nd Ed.
Everything® Get-a-Job Book
Everything® Job Interview Book
Everything® New Teacher Book
Everything® Online Job Search Book
Everything® Paying for College Book
Everything® Practice Interview Book
Everything® Resume Book, 2nd Ed.
Everything® Study Book

SELF-HELP

Everything® Great Sex Book
Everything® Kama Sutra Book
Everything® Self-Esteem Book

SPORTS & FITNESS

Everything® Fishing Book
Everything® Fly-Fishing Book
Everything® Golf Instruction Book

Everything® Pilates Book
Everything® Running Book
Everything® Total Fitness Book
Everything® Weight Training Book
Everything® Yoga Book

TRAVEL

Everything® Family Guide to Hawaii
Everything® Family Guide to New York City, 2nd Ed.
Everything® Family Guide to RV Travel & Campgrounds
Everything® Family Guide to the Walt Disney World Resort®, Universal Studios®, and Greater Orlando, 4th Ed.
Everything® Family Guide to Washington D.C., 2nd Ed.
Everything® Guide to Las Vegas
Everything® Guide to New England
Everything® Travel Guide to the Disneyland Resort®, California Adventure®, Universal Studios®, and the Anaheim Area

WEDDINGS

Everything® Bachelorette Party Book, $9.95
Everything® Bridesmaid Book, $9.95

Everything® Elopement Book, $9.95
Everything® Father of the Bride Book, $9.95
Everything® Groom Book, $9.95
Everything® Mother of the Bride Book, $9.95
Everything® Wedding Book, 3rd Ed.
Everything® Wedding Checklist, $9.95
Everything® Wedding Etiquette Book, $7.95
Everything® Wedding Organizer, $15.00
Everything® Wedding Shower Book, $7.95
Everything® Wedding Vows Book, $7.95
Everything® Weddings on a Budget Book, $9.95

WRITING

Everything® Creative Writing Book
Everything® Get Published Book
Everything® Grammar and Style Book
Everything® Guide to Writing a Book Proposal
Everything® Guide to Writing a Novel
Everything® Guide to Writing Children's Books
Everything® Screenwriting Book
Everything® Writing Poetry Book
Everything® Writing Well Book

. . . .

We have Everything® for the beginner crafter!
All titles are $14.95

Everything® Crafts—Baby Scrapbooking
1-59337-225-6

Everything® Crafts—Bead Your Own Jewelry
1-59337-142-X

Everything® Crafts—Create Your Own Greeting Cards
1-59337-226-4

Everything® Crafts—Easy Projects
1-59337-298-1

Everything® Crafts—Polymer Clay for Beginners
1-59337-230-2

Everything® Crafts—Rubber Stamping Made Easy
1-59337-229-9

Everything® Crafts—Wedding Decorations and Keepsakes
1-59337-227-2

Available wherever books are sold!
To order, call 800-872-5627, or visit us at *www.everything.com*
Everything® and everything.com® are registered trademarks of F+W Publications, Inc.